D1458494

Treating Women with Substance Use Disorders During Pregnancy

A Comprehensive Approach to Caring for Mother and Child

Hendrée E. Jones, Ph.D.[1]

and

Karol Kaltenbach, Ph.D.[2]

[1] RTI International, Research Triangle Park, North Carolina 27709; Department of Psychology, University of North Carolina at Chapel Hill, Chapel Hill, North Carolina 27514; and Departments of Psychiatry and Behavioral Sciences and Obstetrics and Gynecology, School of Medicine, Johns Hopkins University, Baltimore, Maryland 21224

[2] Departments of Pediatrics and Psychiatry and Human Behavior, Jefferson Medical College, Thomas Jefferson University, Philadelphia, Pennsylvania 19107

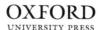

OXFORD
UNIVERSITY PRESS

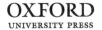

OXFORD
UNIVERSITY PRESS

Oxford University Press is a department of the University of Oxford.
It furthers the University's objective of excellence in research, scholarship,
and education by publishing worldwide.

Oxford   New York
Auckland   Cape Town   Dar es Salaam   Hong Kong   Karachi
Kuala Lumpur   Madrid   Melbourne   Mexico City   Nairobi
New Delhi   Shanghai   Taipei   Toronto

With offices in
Argentina   Austria   Brazil   Chile   Czech Republic   France   Greece
Guatemala   Hungary   Italy   Japan   Poland   Portugal   Singapore
South Korea   Switzerland   Thailand   Turkey   Ukraine   Vietnam

Oxford is a registered trade mark of Oxford University Press in the UK and certain other countries.

Published in the United States of America by
Oxford University Press
198 Madison Avenue, New York, NY 10016

Library of Congress Cataloging-in-Publication Data

Jones, Hendrée E.
    Treating women with substance use disorders during pregnancy: a comprehensive approach to caring for mother
    and child / Hendrée E. Jones and Karol Kaltenbach.
       p.; cm.
    Includes bibliographical references and index.
    ISBN 978-0-19-996855-8 (hardback : alk. paper) – ISBN 978-0-19-996956-2 (ebook)
    I. Kaltenbach, Karol.   II. Title.
    [DNLM: 1. Pregnancy Complications.   2. Substance-Related Disorders – therapy. WM 270]
    LC Classification not assigned
    618.3'68606 – dc23
    2012037225

This material is not intended to be, and should not be considered, a substitute for medical or other professional
advice. Treatment for the conditions described in this material is highly dependent on the individual
circumstances. And, while this material is designed to offer accurate information with respect to the subject
matter covered and to be current as of the time it was written, research and knowledge about medical and health
issues is constantly evolving and dose schedules for medications are being revised continually, with new side effects
recognized and accounted for regularly. Readers must therefore always check the product information and clinical
procedures with the most up-to-date published product information and data sheets provided by the manufacturers
and the most recent codes of conduct and safety regulation. The publisher and the authors make no representations
or warranties to readers, express or implied, as to the accuracy or completeness of this material. Without limiting
the foregoing, the publisher and the authors make no representations or warranties as to the accuracy or efficacy
of the drug dosages mentioned in the material. The authors and the publisher do not accept, and expressly disclaim,
any responsibility for any liability, loss or risk that may be claimed or incurred as a consequence of the use and/or
application of any of the contents of this material.

9 8 7 6 5 4 3 2 1
Printed in the United States of America
on acid-free paper

We dedicate this book to the powerful, beautiful, and strong patients who have shared the innermost corners of their lives with us. Thank you for teaching us about survival, addiction, recovery, and renewal and letting us experience the awe that comes when women find their voice. We are forever grateful for all you have taught us about life, patience, and the promise of human potential.

We gratefully acknowledge our flexible husbands, who have been steadfast supporters of all we do. Thank you for being the roots that ground us. We also are indebted to our children for their sacrifices and unconditional love. You are the greatest gift life brings.

CONTENTS

ACKNOWLEDGMENTS

We would like to take this opportunity to thank the dedicated staff and colleagues of the centers where we work. We are forever indebted to the patients with whom we have had the privilege to work and who have generously shared so much of their lives, struggles, and joys with us. We greatly appreciate the support from the National Institute on Drug Abuse, which enabled us to conduct many of the studies that serve as the foundation of the knowledge we share with you. Finally, we thank our families for their love, patience, sacrifice, and understanding as we worked late evenings, weekends, and holidays to complete this book.

INTRODUCTION

A man approached a young woman on the beach and asked, "Why in the world are you throwing starfish into the water?" "If the starfish stay on the beach, when the tide goes out and the sun rises higher, they will die," replied the young woman as she continued tossing them out to sea. "That's ridiculous! There are thousands of miles of beach and millions of starfish. You can't really believe that what you are doing can possibly make a difference!" The young woman picked up another starfish and said, tossing it into the waves, "It makes a difference to this one."

This story illustrates what many professionals feel as they care for and treat women for substance use disorders during pregnancy. We are often asked, "Isn't that a depressing job?" or "Why would you want to do that?" Sometimes we hear a statement like, "How frustrating that must be to treat those pregnant women. What hope do they have of getting better?" While the reality is that treating women for substance use disorders during pregnancy is a highly demanding challenge, helping these patients make changes in their lives represents some of the most rewarding experiences in our professional lives. This book provides both an overview and an in-depth discussion of the many aspects of a comprehensive care model for the treatment of pregnant women with substance use disorders. The goal is to optimize the rewards that both patients and providers experience during the treatment relationship.

In this introduction we discuss the extent of substance use in pregnant women in the United States. We provide definitions and explain the language used throughout the book, offer a historical perspective on the problem, and conclude with an outline of the goals, audience, and composition of the book.

SUBSTANCE USE DURING PREGNANCY: AN ALARMING PUBLIC HEALTH PROBLEM

Substance use disorders during pregnancy remain an alarming public health problem that is widespread and complex in both its origins and its treatment. It is estimated that among pregnant women in the United States, approximately 16.3% smoked cigarettes, 10.8% drank alcohol, and 4.4% used illicit drugs in the past month (SAMHSA Office of Applied Statistics 2009–2010).

The distinction between legal and illegal substances has led the public to erroneously believe that there is a relationship between the legality of a substance and the severity of its negative impact on fetal and neonatal development and growth. In fact, if substances were ranked in terms of the severity of their devastating consequences to fetal and maternal health, the two legal substances of alcohol and tobacco would likely trump the negative consequences associated with illicit substances like cocaine, opioids, and marijuana. The effects of *in utero* exposure to alcohol include miscarriage; premature delivery; mental retardation; learning, emotional, and behavioral problems; and physical defects of the heart, face, and other organs (SAMHSA, 2007). *In utero* tobacco exposure appears to increase the risk of premature birth and low birth weight, which are risk factors for mortality, morbidity, and developmental problems later in life (CDC, 2007). In contrast, while the scientific and lay communities have given an enormous amount of attention to the risks of *in utero* cocaine exposure, the effects appear more subtle than those of tobacco (Slotkin, 1998). Thus, the assessment and treatment of pregnant women with substance use disorders cannot be focused on the cessation of one substance in isolation because these patients are quite often using multiple substances that may have additive or even synergistic effects on the health and well-being of the mother, fetus, and/or neonate.

While the potential consequences of substance use during pregnancy for the health and well-being of the mother, fetus, and neonate are concerning, substance use during pregnancy must be viewed in context and in relation to multiple other factors that can compromise healthy pregnancies. Women who use substances during pregnancy often do so in the context of intricately complex individual, social, and environmental factors, including a history of childhood trauma, poor nutrition, extreme stress, violence of multiple forms, poor housing conditions, exposure to environmental toxins and diseases, and depression, which can all affect postnatal outcomes (Robins & Mills, 1993). While the odds are often stacked against women who use substances during pregnancy, each patient is unique and must be viewed in the context of her own risk and protective factors to optimize her treatment and outcomes for herself and her child.

LANGUAGE AND TERMS USED THROUGHOUT THE BOOK

We deliberately chose to use several terms throughout the book. First, the term "substance use disorder" has been used to indicate the spectrum of problems with substances for which pregnant women are treated. We selected this term because it is both a scientific term and accepted nomenclature that encompasses the widest spectrum of problem substance use, which includes use that does not meet the criteria for abuse (a recurring pattern of alcohol or other substance use that impairs a person's functioning in one or more important life areas) or dependence (a primary chronic disease with genetic, psychological, and environmental factors influencing its development and manifestations), as well as both substance abuse and substance dependence. We have avoided the term "addiction" (continued use of a substance despite its detrimental effects, compromised control over the use of a substance, preoccupation with wanting to feel the substance's effects, and significant quantities of time involved in activities to obtain the substance) and the phrase "addicted during pregnancy" due to their lack of specificity and because they tend to carry forward into the discussion of the infant—and the infant is then incorrectly labeled as addicted. In the few instances where the term "substance use disorders" was not used, we did so to be consistent with the literature that was being cited.

Second, the phrase or variant of the phrase "treating women for substance use disorders during pregnancy" or "pregnant women in treatment for a substance abuse disorder" may seem wordy. However, we chose to do so to emphasize that the substance use disorder almost always precedes the pregnancy. And of course, we want to emphasize that it is the patient who is being treated, not the substance use disorder itself.

Third, we chose to use the word "patient" rather than "client." Yes, some see the term "patient" as a label that creates a power differential between the patient and provider, in favor of the provider. But to the best of our knowledge, there are no data to support the use of one word over the other in terms of outcomes for the treatment of substance use disorders.

Finally, we use the word "provider" because it can indicate not only a clinician but anyone who is providing a service to or for the patient.

HISTORICAL CONTEXT OF TREATING SUBSTANCE USE DISORDERS DURING PREGNANCY

Use of substances is so common in almost all cultures that it appears to be a basic human activity. Because substances are so intertwined with many people's fears and desires, it is difficult to provide neutral information on this topic.

Moreover, when discussing substance use, no condition inspires more emotion and controversy than substance use during pregnancy. This has been an important health issue in the United States for centuries. For example, in the 1800s, 66% to 75% of individuals with opium substance use disorders were women. The most common source of opium for women was medical prescriptions to treat pain (Kandall, 1996). During the late 1800s physicians recognized the neonatal opioid withdrawal syndrome and the need to treat with morphine the newborns of mothers who had taken opium during pregnancy in order to prevent morbidity and mortality (Earle, 1888).

By the 1900s physicians were becoming better educated about the drawbacks of prescribing narcotics, and legitimate supplies of narcotics then shrank. As a result, women unable to stop using substances were forced to seek them from illegitimate sources. Passage of the Harrison Narcotic Act of 1914 greatly changed narcotic prescribing and dispensing practices—for example, addictive substances now needed to be prescribed by a licensed health professional. While some enlightened physicians treated opioid use disorders with morphine, in 1919 this practice was prohibited by the Supreme Court. The result of this decision was the segregation of the treatment of substance use disorders from general medical practice (Kandall, 1996).

In the 1960s and 1970s, substance use became an important social issue, in part due to the high rates of opioid use disorders among returning Vietnam veterans and the increasing volume of voices from advocates for women's health and social equality. In the 1970s, the National Institute on Drug Abuse (NIDA) started projects to address substance use among women, especially pregnant women (Kandall, 1996). For example, NIDA's "Perinatal 20" project in the 1980s and 1990s focused on the special needs of pregnant and postpartum women using crack and cocaine.

During the 1980s the "War on Drugs" was at its height and the media proclaimed a "crack baby" epidemic. News stories cast these children as damaged and unable to learn, and the mothers of these children were portrayed as selfish and unloving. The reports of "crack babies" fueled the most punitive strategy toward substance-using pregnant women to date: the prosecution of pregnant women under a variety of state laws involving assault with a deadly weapon, delivery of a controlled substance to a minor, and child abuse (Paltrow, 1990). Unfortunately, history is repeating itself with the recent media attention sensationalizing the increased prenatal exposure to prescription opioids (e.g., Curtis, 2012). While it is understandable that many individuals have argued in favor of controlling a woman's behavior to protect her fetus, the result has been to transform pregnant women into criminals, punishable by law for making poor choices. Pregnant women seeking help for their substance use disorder do so in this context of extreme emotion and stigma.

While stigma exists for men and nonpregnant women who use substances, no other group of substance-using adults are likely subjected to more stigma than are women who consume both legal and illegal substances during pregnancy. This stigmatization is exacerbated by emotion-driven opinions that substance use always results in poor parenting and that substance-using mothers are unable and unwilling to care for their infants. Yet a large body of research has found that women who use substances can be adequate parents (Buchanan & Young, 2002; Colten, 1980; Leeders, 1992; Sterk-Elifson, 1996; Sowder & Burt, 1980).

OUTLINE OF THE BOOK

Our goal in developing this book was to create a resource for several audiences. The first is professionals who encounter on a daily basis women with substance use disorders who are also pregnant. These professionals include psychologists, psychiatrists, social workers, obstetricians, family practice physicians, and counselors. Second, this book will serve as a valuable resource for neonatologists, pediatricians, nurses, allied health professionals, mental health care practitioners, and pastoral counselors. While all levels of providers may benefit from the material, this book is aimed at providing state-of-the-science information to in-training, trained, and practicing providers in many different disciplines.

This book aims to provide the first-ever in-depth comprehensive and evidence-based overview of the treatment of women with substance use disorders while they are pregnant. The book provides readers with information that will not only aid them in identifying, assessing, and understanding the issues involved in this population but will also provide practical tools to implement the clinical recommendations and best practices that are supported by the research literature and clinical experience from a comprehensive care program that specializes in treating women for substance use disorders during pregnancy. This book is designed to be a standalone guide covering all aspects of treatment a provider needs to know when faced with caring for a woman with a substance use disorder during pregnancy. Moreover, the book is intended to be accessible yet scholarly. We include chapters on all aspects related to the understanding and treatment of women with substance use disorders during pregnancy. We did not want to write either a "how-to" case example manual or an exhaustive review of the literature. Rather, we have tried to strike a balance between the best scientific information and reasoned clinical wisdom to fill in where evidence-based information is absent and to convey this information in a form that is practical and accessible.

There are three sections to the book. Section I encompasses the ethical and legal issues faced by the patient and provider (Chapter 1), the theories and concepts that underlie the treatment of women with substance use disorders during pregnancy (Chapter 2), and the importance of the overall context in which treatment is provided (Chapter 3). Section II discusses the identification of substance use disorders in pregnant patients (Chapter 4), the comprehensive assessment of these patients (Chapter 5), and the individualized care plan that should be developed, initiated, monitored, and completed (Chapter 6). Section III covers methods to assist patients in stabilizing and withdrawing from substances (Chapter 7), the approaches that are available to care for the dually diagnosed patient (Chapter 8), the obstetrical aspects of care in this population (Chapter 9), and how to assist the patient in caring for her substance-exposed newborn (Chapter 10). Chapter 11, which covers treatment programming, discusses group and individual therapy topics and objective methods for verifying abstinence from substances and ways to address relapse. Chapter 12, which reviews trauma-informed treatment, discusses methods for helping patients heal from past trauma and minimize future trauma exposure. Chapter 13, on case management, covers social service aspects such as housing, transportation, parenting, employment, education, finances, and legal assistance. The contents of the entire book are brought together in Chapter 14 with a practical discussion of how to develop a comprehensive care program.

CONCLUSION

This book is in many ways a compilation of the knowledge, research, and practical experience that we have gained during our careers in treating women with substance use disorders during pregnancy, together with the attendant clinical research in this area. One of the most important messages of this book is that treating patients with substance use disorders during pregnancy represents a short and finite duration during which we can begin to address the multiple, intersecting, and complex issues that led to substance use initiation and continuation in the patient. For the vast majority of pregnant women seeking treatment for substance use disorders, substance use started long before they became pregnant, so it is unrealistic to expect that such a complex and entrenched problem will be alleviated in a few weeks or even months. However, pregnancy is a sensitive time during which a woman can enter treatment and begin to make important steps on the path to recovery of functioning as a complete and fulfilled person in her many roles as mother, daughter, partner, friend, coworker, and community citizen.

REFERENCES

Buchanan, J., & Young, L. (2002). Child protection: social worker's views. In H. Klee, M. Jackson, & S. Lewis (Eds.), *Drug misuse and motherhood* (pp. 195–210). London: Routledge.

Centers for Disease ControlPrevention (CDC). (2007). *Smoking and tobacco fact sheet: women and smoking.*

Colten, M. A. (1980). *Comparison of heroin-addicted and non-addicted mothers: Their attitudes, beliefs, and parenting experiences, Heroin-addicted parents and their children: Two reports.* National Institute on Drug Abuse Services Research Report, U.S. Department of Health and Human Services; Public Health Service; Alcohol, Drug Abuse, and Mental Health Administration, Washington, DC, pp. 1–18.

Curtis, W. (July 9, 2012). Innocent victims: Drug dependence begins early for some Mainers. *Kennebec Journal*, Augusta, Maine.

Earle, F. B. (1888). Maternal opium habit and infant mortality. *Medical Standards, 111,* 2–4.

Kandall, S. R. (1996). *Substance and shadow: Women and addiction in the United States.* Cambridge, MA: Harvard University Press

Leeders, F. (1992). Drug-addicted parents and their children. *International Journal of Drug Policy, 3*(4), 204–210.

Paltrow, L. M. (1990). When becoming pregnant is a crime. *Criminal Justice Ethics, 9,* 41–47.

Robins, L. N., & Mills, J. L. (1993). Effects of in utero exposure to street drugs. *American Journal of Public Health, 83*(Suppl.), 1–32.

Slotkin, T. A. (1998). Fetal nicotine or cocaine exposure: which one is worse? *Journal of Pharmacology and Experimental Therapeutics, 285*(3), 931–945.

Sowder, B., & Burt, M. (1980). Children of addicts and nonaddicts: A comparative investigation in five urban sites. In *Heroin-addicted parents and their children* (DHHS publications no. ADM 81–1028) (pp. 19–35). Rockville, MD: National Institute on Drug Abuse.

Sterk-Elifson, C. (1996). Just for fun? Cocaine use among middle-class women. *Journal of Drug Issues, 26,* 63–76.

SAMHSA Office of Applied Statistics. Results from the 2010 National Survey on Drug Use and Health: Summary of National Findings. http://www.samhsa.gov/data/NSDUH/2k10NSDUH/2k10Results.htm (accessed December 19, 2012).

Substance Abuse and Mental Health Services Administration, U.S. Department of Health and Human Services. (2007). *Fetal alcohol spectrum disorders.*

Overview of Macro-Level Issues to Consider When Treating Women for Substance Use Disorders During Pregnancy

1

Legal and Ethical Issues in Providing Treatment to Women with Substance Use Disorders During Pregnancy

OVERVIEW

In this chapter we discuss a number of legal issues involved in providing treatment to women with substance use disorders during pregnancy, including attempts to prosecute pregnant women on such charges as distribution of drugs to minors and interpreting child abuse statutes as applicable to the fetus. We examine the Federal Child Abuse Prevention and Treatment Act (CAPTA) and states that have enacted legislation and/or expanded their child welfare statutes to include substance use during pregnancy as child abuse or neglect. We describe the issues surrounding the role of substance use disorder treatment providers as mandated reporters of child abuse and/or neglect and potential conflicts that may arise as a result of this mandate and offer suggestions about how to ensure the safety of the child while maintaining support for the mother. We also discuss federal and state regulations regarding the need to maintain the confidentiality of all individuals seeking and entering treatment for a substance use disorder and the practical implications for treatment providers.

INTRODUCTION

There are a number of legal and ethical issues that may either directly or indirectly affect the delivery of services to women with substance use disorders during pregnancy. Pregnant women with substance use disorders are often

subjected to prejudicial and judgmental treatment, not only by health care providers, but by reinterpretation of existing child abuse statues in which a fetus is
considered a child. Moreover, coercive policies may be implemented by child
welfare systems and juvenile/family court. In the extreme, some of these actions
ignore constitutional protections, and, at the least, deter women from seeking prenatal care and treatment for their substance use disorders. Underlying
these actions is the spurious assumption that if faced with the threat of incarceration or losing their child(ren), they will simply stop using drugs. Such an
approach ignores or does not recognize the nature of substance use disorders.
This approach considers a substance use disorder a moral failure or a lack of
individual willpower rather than a serious life-threatening illness. Paramount
to addressing these issues is the understanding that pregnant women with
substance use disorders are women with substance use disorders who become
pregnant, with all of the complex problems associated with substance use
disorders. This is a critical distinction that has significant impact on meeting
the needs of this at-risk population.

STATUTORY ACTIONS DIRECTED AT WOMEN WITH
SUBSTANCE USE DISORDERS DURING PREGNANCY

As discussed in the Introduction, in the United States we can trace the emergence of publicly supported treatment programs for pregnant women with substance use disorders to the early 1970s, with such programs primarily directed
to opioid use disorders. A number of these programs were research-based and
identified the need for and value of specialized comprehensive treatment for
pregnant women with substance use disorders (see Chapter 5). However, in
the late 1980s, as the cocaine epidemic swept across the country, there was
a media frenzy focused on the cocaine-using pregnant woman and the outcome for her child. The term "crack baby" carried prejudices and fear with
the expectation that this child was irredeemably harmed. The result was that
lawmakers and public policy officials dismissed the value of substance use
treatment and turned to the judicial system to address the "problem." Harsh
legal measures against pregnant women with substance use disorders began
to be implemented. Anti-drug distribution laws and "fetal abuse" statutes, in
which existing child abuse statutes were extended to include the conduct of
women during the prenatal period, were frequently used to prosecute pregnant women for substance use (Scott, 2006). In these cases, the fetus was determined to be a "child," so pregnant women were arrested for possession of a
controlled substance and delivering drugs to a minor, and/or charged with
child endangerment or abuse.

The most notorious of these efforts was a policy established at the public hospital at the Medical University of South Carolina (MUSC). In 1989, the hospital began to routinely order urine drug screenings of maternity patients, initially referring anyone who tested positive to treatment for substance use. However, within the year, after learning that the police in Greensville, SC, were arresting pregnant women who used cocaine on the theory that such use harmed the fetus and therefore constituted child abuse, the hospital offered to identify and assist in the prosecution of pregnant women who used cocaine. The end result was police apprehending some patients within hours of giving birth and transporting them to jail in handcuffs and leg shackles. There was even the more extreme case of a women handcuffed to her bed during delivery. Ten women who had positive urine drug screening results and were subsequently arrested brought suit against the hospital and the city. The jury found in favor of the hospital and city but ultimately, in 2001, the U.S. Supreme Court ruled in favor of the women in *Ferguson v. the City of Charlestown, SC* (2001), based on the determination that the women did not consent to drug testing, which violated their Fourth Amendment right to be free from unreasonable search and seizures.

Admittedly the MUSC case was an extreme action; however, as late as 2000 over 200 women in 30 states had been prosecuted for fetal abuse because of their substance use disorder (Paltrow et al., 2000). During this time eight states considered but failed to pass legislation that would make it a crime to have a substance use disorder during pregnancy. Currently no state has a criminal law in which it is a crime to use an illicit substance while pregnant. However, prosecutors have used existing criminal laws to charge pregnant women with a wide range of crimes, such as possession of a controlled substance, delivering drugs to a minor, assault with a deadly weapon, manslaughter, and child abuse and neglect (Guttmacher Institute, 2000). Although most such convictions have been overturned on appeal, the South Carolina State Supreme Court has upheld that the fetus is a person under the state's criminal child endangerment act (Ketteringham et al., 2011), and there is a case before the Alabama Supreme Court challenging the broad interpretation of the 2006 chemical endangerment law written to protect children from the dangers of methamphetamine labs that is being used to prosecute women who give birth to infants prenatally exposed to illicit substances (Alcoholism Drug Abuse Weekly, 2012).

In efforts to respond to the risks associated with illicit substance use by pregnant women, a number of states have expanded their civil child welfare requirements to include prenatal drug exposure. As of this writing, 15 states define substance use during pregnancy as child abuse, and three of the 15 also authorize civil commitment (e.g., forced admission to an inpatient treatment program) (Guttmacher Institute, 2012). Up-to-date information about state policies in regard to substance use by pregnant women can be found at www.guttmacher.org

Another valuable resource is the Child Welfare Information Gateway, Children's Bureau/ACYF, DHHS, which maintains information on state laws that address substance use by parents within child protection statutes (see www.childwelfare.gov).

In addition to variability in legislation among states are the intra- and interstate differences in response to the federal Child Abuse Prevention and Treatment Act (CAPTA). Initially enacted in 1974 to provide funding to states in support of child protective service agencies, it was amended in 2003, requiring states to have policies for notifying child protective services of newborns exposed to illicit substances *in utero* and establishing a plan of care for newborns affected by illicit substance use or withdrawal symptoms resulting from prenatal drug exposure (Child Welfare Information Gateway, 2009). There is considerable variability in the manner in which states have responded to CAPTA. For example, states have amended their civil welfare statues (as described in the previous paragraph), changed their interpretation of reporting requirements, and/or redefined withdrawal (i.e., from illicit substance use or as a result of prescribed medication). Making the situation even more complicated is the fact that there is often considerable variability from county to county as to how the federal law is interpreted, especially in terms of prenatal exposure to methadone used in maternal treatment for opioid dependence. For example, in one county in New Jersey, the Department of Youth and Family Services (DYFS) works closely with opioid treatment programs so that decisions to remove an infant from a mother's custody will take into account how well the mother is doing in treatment, whereas in another New Jersey county, engagement in treatment is not taken into account and mothers receiving methadone treatment often have to go to court to retain custody of their newborns.

While it might be argued that drastic measures are necessary to ensure the safety of the child, it is essential that any such actions are based on scientific evidence, not presumptions or political posturing. The MUSC case previously cited provides an example in which there was no scientific evidence to support the actions that were taken. Indeed, there are no data to support the position that every child exposed to cocaine is harmed by such exposure (Frank et al., 2001), and the punitive measures employed in this case have been shown to have an effect exactly opposite to that which was intended (Gellman, 2000). Such actions ignore the nature of substance use disorders, overlook the complex array of problems associated with it that can be exacerbated during pregnancy (see Chapter 5), and threaten the well-being of the fetus because they deter women from seeking the necessary prenatal care and substance use disorder treatment (Gellman, 2000). Unfortunately, such prejudicial and destructive actions are often the result of a district attorney in an election year who wants to make maternal substance use a campaign issue.

These legal challenges make it incumbent upon individuals who provide treatment to pregnant women with substance use disorders to advocate for the dignity and right of the woman to seek and receive treatment and to provide the support she needs to be successful in her recovery and in her role as a mother while at the same time maintaining balance with the requirement of mandated reporting if the child is in fact at risk for abuse and/or neglect.

MANDATED REPORTERS

The fact that treatment providers are mandated by law to report any incident of child abuse and/or neglect often creates a tension between the patient and the treatment program. It is important that this issue be addressed openly and directly when the patient is admitted to treatment so that feelings of betrayal do not occur if such reporting becomes necessary. During the intake process, the patient should have a clear understanding that the program will provide support and assistance with her caregiving responsibilities, but that the program has a legal responsibility to report if there is concern for the safety and well-being of her child(ren). If a situation develops that requires reporting, the patient should be informed of the fact, be given clear reasons why the report is necessary, and be provided with the support and direction needed to address/resolve the situation. Interventions and strategies to eliminate risk to the child should be incorporated within her treatment plan (see Chapter 6), and therapeutic intervention should be provided to address anger and loss issues and risks of relapse. Consent should be obtained for her counselor and/or case manager to speak with the child protection case worker in order to assist her in negotiating and responding to the child protection system appropriately. Additional services such as family therapy, referral to community legal services, etc. should be provided when warranted. The patient needs to understand that concern and support for her and assistance in addressing her needs are not diminished by the need to involve protective services for the child.

PROTECTION OF CONFIDENTIALITY

The confidentiality of all patient information pertaining to enrollment in a treatment program for substance use is protected under federal stature 42 CFR Part 2 (relating to confidentiality of alcohol and substance use patient records). The purpose of these regulations is to protect patients who are attending treatment programs for a substance use disorder, specifically that they do not become vulnerable due to the availability of their patient records. The regulations impose severe restrictions upon the disclosure and use of patient records. In addition to the federal regulations, state drug and alcohol divisions have their own regulations. The foundation for these regulations is that patients are entitled to the expectation that information about them will be treated with respect and confidentiality. It recognizes that such confidentiality is a necessary component for patients to access and engage in treatment. While the importance of these regulations is well appreciated, the limitations imposed may cause tension between other agencies, such as child protective services, courts, third-party payers, etc. For example, child protective services may seek to determine if a mother has relapsed, the results of her urine drug screens, what medications and dose she is receiving, and whether she is compliant with care. Not only can no information be disclosed without the written consent of a patient, any answer to a request for information must be made in such a way that will not reveal that an individual has been or is currently being treated for alcohol or substance use. This restriction requires that all staff be well trained in confidentiality and be adept at parrying adamant requesters. It is helpful to have a script for staff to follow so that even when well intentioned they do not indirectly confirm that an individual is a patient.

Confidentiality restrictions apply to parents, family members, and partners, even to such innocuous requests to confirm when the patient should be ready to be picked up. It also applies to all visitors to the program, including friends, professionals, auditors, etc. Any person entering the program should sign a confidentiality statement that he or she will not disclose the identity of any patient or patient-related information that he or she may obtain while on the premises.

Signed consent forms need to be included for any exchange of information, including program physicians communicating with primary care physicians, sharing information with other treatment programs in the case of arranging for transfers, and providing medication information (e.g., methadone dose to prison health systems for incarcerated patients).

The authority of the court can be intimidating, and it is not unusual for a subpoena to arrive, often at the last minute, for a counselor to appear in court in regard to a proceeding involving one of his or her patients. Staff members need to be well versed in the confidentiality regulations because they supersede a subpoena in that a duly executed court order is required to compel disclosure of information without patient consent.

Additional tensions often occur between treatment programs and third-party payers. While certain information can be released to a third-party payer to determine the necessity for admission, continued stay, concurrent reviews, etc., the content of the information is limited. This restriction can place providers in the difficult position of refusing to release requested information to the payer. It is important that all parties understand the limitations imposed by the regulations, and when there is discordance between regulations and payer expectations, it may be best addressed by involving the state department/division for drug and alcohol services.

SUMMARY

Treatment providers must be aware of the prejudicial legal ramifications that pregnant women with substance use disorders often face. They should not only provide advocacy for their patients but take an active role in educating community leaders and political representatives about the nature of substance use disorders and the complex array of issues that are characteristic of pregnant women with substance use disorders so that efforts and resources are directed at services rather than criminalization. A delicate balance must be achieved to ensure that the best interests of both mother and child are met, with the understanding that the safety of the child is paramount. All staff and program policies must reflect a through knowledge of confidentiality regulations so that no patient information is ever disclosed without patient consent unless allowed by law.

REFERENCES

Alcoholism Drug Abuse Weekly (March 19, 2012). 24(12), Available online: ISSN 1556–7591, www.wileyonlinelibrary.com (accessed July 3, 2012).

Child Welfare Information Gateway (2009). Parental drug use as child abuse: summary of state laws. Available online: www.childwelfare.gov (accessed July 3, 2012).

Ferguson v. City of Charleston, 532 U.S. 67, 85–86 (2001) 42 CFR Part 2, Chapter 1 Public Health Service, Department of Health and Human Services Part 2 Confidentiality of Alcohol and Drug Abuse Patient Records.

Frank, D. A., Augustyn, M., Knight, W. G., Pell, T., & Zuckerman, B. (2001). Growth, development, and behavior in early childhood following prenatal cocaine exposure: a systematic review. *Journal of the American Medical Association*, 285(12), 1613–1625.

Gellman, S. Brief *Amici Curiae* in support of Appellants Brief re Baby Boy Blackshears. 90 Ohio St. 3b 197, 2000-Ohio-173.

Guttmacher Institute (December 2000). State responses to substance abuse among pregnant women. Available online: www.guttmacher.org (accessed July 6, 2012).

Guttmacher Institute (July 1, 2012). State policies in brief: substance use during pregnancy. Available online: www.guttmacher.org (accessed July 6, 2012).

Ketteringham, E. S., Korn, A., & Paltrow, L. M. (2011). Proposition 26: The cost to all women. *Mississippi Law Journal,* 81 Supra 81.

Paltrow, L., Cohen, D., & Carey, C. (2000). *Year 2000 Overview: Governmental responses to pregnant women who use alcohol and other drugs.* Joint document produced by the Women's Law Project, Philadelphia, PA, and National Advocates for Pregnant Women, New York.

Scott, T. (2006). Repercussions of the crack baby epidemic: why a message of care rather than punishment is needed for pregnant drug-users. *National Black Law Journal, 19*(2), 203–221.

2

Basic Theories and Concepts Guiding the Treatment of Substance Use Disorders in Pregnant Women

OVERVIEW

This chapter builds upon the Introduction, which provided an overview of the history of treating women for substance use disorders during pregnancy and introduced key terms that are used through this chapter and the remainder of the book. This chapter continues the discussion begun in Chapter 1 of treatment for substance use disorders in pregnant women by introducing the theoretical principles that underlie the treatments driving effective results.

In this chapter we review the key concepts and theories that serve as the foundation for the treatment of substance use disorders in the pregnant patient. First, we discuss key theories underlying many effective treatments for substance use disorders, including behavioral learning theories, cognitive learning theories, and social learning theory. Second, we present key concepts such as a review of substance use as a motivated behavior and motivational constructs relevant to substance use. Next, we give examples of specific behavioral approaches to highlight the implementation of these theories as applied in practice. Finally, we emphasize key points made in the chapter.

INTRODUCTION

The key theories and concepts providing the foundation for the most prominent treatments of substance use disorders are summarized in the present chapter. We provide examples of how these theories and concepts inform and are applied in the approaches to treatment of substance use disorders during pregnancy. It is recognized that the vast majority of pregnant women are treated with a creative melding of treatment approaches that are sometimes, but not always, based on an understanding on the part of the treatment provider of the principles and theories underlying various approaches to treatment. The material in this chapter is presented to illuminate for the treatment provider the rationale and most recent evidence in support of the use of effective treatments with the pregnant population diagnosed with substance use disorders.

Before we review the key theories and concepts forming the foundation of the most effective substance use disorder treatments, it is important to make the point that substance use disorders are motivated behaviors and neither a moral failing nor purely a physical disease. The fact that substance use disorders represent motivated behaviors is critically important for understanding how to treat these types of disorders. When treating patients with substance use disorders, the provider is focused on helping the patient modify her thought processes and belief structures as well as her external environments to gain control over how she is behaving. This perspective differs from what other providers do when treating more physically based diseases such as certain cancers, where the treatment focuses on curing the disease by, for example, removing the diseased part of the body. Unfortunately, there are no "cures" for substance use disorders—yet there are some very effective treatments that are based on the principles of behavioral theories that are presented below. This is an important distinction: the goal of substance use treatment is not to "cure" the disease but to facilitate the patient in extinguishing her responses to environmental cues that set the occasion for substance use, helping her shape her behavior so that substance use behaviors become incompatible with new behaviors associated with a different way of living life and continue behaviors whose consequences effectively compete with substance use. While medications can certainly be effective for some substance use disorders (e.g., methadone and buprenorphine to treat opioid dependence), the use of medication should serve to stabilize the patient so she can focus on the full spectrum of treatment components. Thus, medication can serve as a foundation on which to build treatment rather than the treatment itself.

KEY THEORIES UNDERLYING ANY SUBSTANCE USE DISORDER TREATMENTS, INCLUDING THOSE FOR PREGNANT WOMEN

Succinctly, the foundation of all behavioral treatments for substance use disorders can be traced back to three learning theories.

Behaviorist learning theories

The theory of behaviorism is most often associated with B. F. Skinner, who put forth four tenets of learning: (1) learning is demonstrated by a change in behavior; (2) the environment plays a primary role in shaping behavior; (3) the principle of contiguity (how close in time two events must be for a bond to be formed); and (4) the principle of reinforcement (increasing the likelihood that an event will be repeated) (Skinner, 1971). For behaviorists, learning a new behavior occurs through conditioning. There are two types of conditioning, classical and operant.

In classical conditioning, behavior becomes a reflex response to a stimulus. For example, if a person repeatedly eats hamburgers at a fast-food restaurant and sees the sign of the fast-food restaurant before and while she is eating the hamburger, eventually the sign of the fast-food restaurant itself will cause her mouth to water without eating the hamburger.

With operant conditioning, behaviors are shaped by their consequences. This means that behaviors are shaped by the reinforcement (reward or a punishment) after the behavior occurs. A behavior may result either in reinforcement, which increases the likelihood of recurrence of the behavior, or punishment, which decreases the likelihood of recurrence of the behavior. However, a punisher is not considered to be punishment if it does not result in the reduction of the behavior: the terms "punishment" and "reinforcement" are determined only as a result of the actions of the person in response to the punishment or reinforcement. Within this framework, behaviorists are particularly interested in measurable changes in behavior. It is important to note that not all behavioral disorders derive from misguided learning. In many ways much of substance use treatment, including treatment for pregnant women, commonly uses punishment and reinforcement. For example, pregnant patients in treatment programs may be "punished" for providing a drug-positive urine sample. The consequences that are aimed at stopping substance use behavior include increasing the treatment intensity and/or the duration of the treatment. Another consequence includes a report to a probation or parole or child protective services about her behavior. Reinforcement of drug abstinence behavior is also used in treatment settings. For example, opioid-dependent pregnant women in treatment for substance dependence can earn take-home methadone doses for providing consistent drug-negative urine samples.

Cognitive Learning Theories

A cognitive learning theory was first proposed by Edward Chace Tolman, who suggested that learning involves central constructs and new ways of perceiving events on the part of the person. This theory relates to cognitive therapy (discussed below) in that it proposes that problems such as substance use disorders are the result of maladaptive ways of thinking, distorted attitudes, and misperceptions of oneself and others (Gross, 1992). An example of when cognitive learning theory is applied in the treatment of pregnant women with substance use disorders is found in group treatments where the focus is on prompting patients to see the more positive side of situations, to help them have a more accurate appraisal of themselves and others, and to change their way of thinking to better cope with stressful situations.

Social Learning Theory

Social learning theory has been considered a transition between behaviorist learning theories and cognitive learning theories. This theory focuses on learning that occurs within a social context. It was first proposed by N. E. Miller and J. Dollard in 1941. They put forth the idea that if one were motivated to learn a behavior, then that behavior would be learned through observing others. By imitating these observed actions, the person would learn the action and would be rewarded with positive reinforcement (Miller & Dollard, 1941). Albert Bandura expanded this theory by asserting that people learn from each other through observation, modeling, and imitation (Ormrod, 1999).

OBSERVATION
People learn by observing the behavior of others and the outcomes of the behaviors that others display. Unlike behaviorist learning theories, social learning theory states that learning can occur without a change in behavior when people learn through observation. Thus, learning may or may not result in behavioral change.

MODELING
Many aspects of behaviors can be learned through modeling. Examples related to substance treatment might include patients watching other patients remain substance-free on a daily basis and patients watching the provider acting with respect and accurate empathy toward other patients as well as the patient herself.

Modeling behavior can result in the teaching and learning of new behavior, as in the case of substance use treatment, when new ways of remaining abstinent can be taught. Modeling can also influence how often previously learned behaviors are performed. For example, in substance use treatment, modeling drug-abstinence behaviors can reduce the frequency with which substance use behavior is exhibited. Modeling can also increase the likelihood that other similar behaviors will be more frequently displayed. For example, in a substance use treatment program, a patient dependent on alcohol might observe a peer attending Narcotics Anonymous meetings and then might start attending Alcoholic Anonymous meetings herself.

IMITATION

Both harmful and healthy behaviors can be learned by imitating the actions of others. For example, individuals can learn to smoke cigarettes by observing and imitating the actions of their favorite movie stars whom they see smoking cigarettes in movies. Healthy behaviors such as abstinence-related behaviors that are shown in substance use treatment can also be learned through imitating the behaviors of others, including peers and providers.

Other aspects of the social learning theory include *self-efficacy* and *self-regulation*. Self-efficacy suggests that people will be more likely to engage in behaviors when they believe they are capable of emitting them successfully. Thus, in substance use treatment, providers often try to help patients increase their belief and confidence in themselves that they will be able to remain abstinent and perform other behaviors (e.g., obtain employment) that will support that abstinence. Self-regulation is when a person chooses her actions based on her own individual thoughts about what is appropriate or inappropriate behavior. In substance use treatment, a great deal of effort is devoted to teaching patients how to increase their self-regulatory behaviors. One way that self-regulation is taught in substance use treatment is by providing rewards to oneself after completing a task. For example, a patient may complete three job applications and then reward herself by taking a warm bubble bath.

Julian B. Rotter advanced social learning theory by integrating learning and personality theories in a novel way that has had an enduring but underrecognized impact on the field of clinical psychology. Rotter posited that individuals are motivated by stimulation. Specifically, they will display behavior in an effort to experience pleasant stimulation and escape or avoid uncomfortable stimulation. The unique aspects of Rotter's social learning theory included the belief that the individual's dynamic interaction with the environment created and maintained his or her personality. Thus, to fully understand a person's behavior, one must consider both what the individual brings to the situation and what the person is noticing and responding to in the environment (http://psych.fullerton.edu/jmearns/rotter.htm). Rotter was an important and undervalued contributor to the cognitive-behavioral therapies used to treat substance use disorders that are discussed below. He viewed maladaptive behaviors, such as substance use, as learned behaviors that individuals come to rely on as their only means of positive stimulation because they have failed to learn a more diverse range of adaptive behaviors to provide them with positive stimulation. Viewing substance use as a maladaptive learned behavior suggests that treatment should teach patients new, more adaptive behaviors to provide positive stimulation.

Another important aspect of Rotter's social learning theory central to understanding and modifying behavior is the concept of expectancies. An individual who has a low expectancy for reward after displaying a certain behavior will expect that the behaviors he or she generates will not be successful in providing positive stimulation or avoiding negative experiences that would determine his or her behavioral response to a stimulus. This low expectation causes the individual to make only a minimal effort to seek the desired experience. Rotter suggested that making only a minimal effort increases the failure opportunities and that these failure experiences in turn reinforce the lack of effort put forth to obtain a given reward. This low threshold for cessation of activity that might take effort to achieve a positive experience or avoid a negative one is often seen in patients with substance use disorders. Thus, using Rotter's theory, a patient exhibiting low expectancies for changing substance use behaviors would be treated by the provider using methods focused on raising the patient's confidence that she can achieve a desired result with more effort. Having the patient make small steps toward the larger goal and experiencing the positive stimulation provided by the achievement of the small goals may help raise her expectancies for future behaviors to provide positive or avoid negative stimulation (Rotter, 1982). For example, a pregnant patient may be first asked to agree to 24 hours of drug abstinence. At the end of the 24 hours, if she is still abstinent she would be highly praised and then asked to agree to 48 hours of abstinence. This chain of small successes may serve to build up her expectations that she can sustain her abstinence for a longer and longer duration each time.

A final aspect that is important to Rotter's social learning theory is the value individuals place on reinforcers. For Rotter, reinforcers are the goals an individual seeks to obtain or attain in his or her life. He argued that individuals with maladaptive behaviors have a mismatch between their desired goals and the realistic goals they can achieve without experiencing multiple failures, thereby leading to low expectancies. Thus, as described above, setting smaller, more appropriately attainable goals is one of several keys to health adaptive behaviors.

In summary, social learning theory posits that behavior is shaped by the understanding that the person has about the relationship between the behavior and the receipt of the reward or punishment, as well as the value that he or she places on that reward or punishment. Social learning theory emphasizes the choice that emitting a behavior represents, whereas operant conditioning theory sees behavior as a reaction based on past consequences of actions.

The above theories, alone or in combination, have been used in the treatment of substance use disorders in pregnant women—often without the explicit recognition that these theories are being applied as part of the treatment process. This lack of recognition may stem from the fact that the theories are complex and necessarily broad. Thus, psychological theories often require translational approaches or practical bridging between theory and everyday clinical practice to allow for their effective use in treatment.

The next section of this chapter will review examples of key concepts that have also helped to shape the current state of substance use disorder treatment for pregnant women.

KEY CONCEPTS INFLUENCING ANY SUBSTANCE USE DISORDER TREATMENTS, INCLUDING THOSE TREATMENTS FOR PREGNANT WOMEN

Behavior as Orderly or Disorderly

The continuum of behavior is anchored by orderly behavior and disorderly behavior. Behaviors are placed along this continuum based on the values and context of the society and groups of individuals in which the behaviors occur. Behaviors, orderly or disorderly, can be viewed from multiple perspectives: physiology, conditioned learning, the value placed on that behavior in society, the expectations about behavior in society, and choice within the confines of culture (McHugh & Slavney, 1998). Where a behavior falls along the continuum can be defined as such by the *methods* used to reach the goal. For example, getting to sleep by relying on sleeping pills is an ordinary goal fulfilled in a maladaptive way. A behavior may be labeled as disorderly as a result of the *consequences* it may bring. For example, an HIV-negative woman having unprotected sexual relations with a HIV-positive partner is an ordinary behavior with dangerous consequences. The *force* with which a behavior is emitted can also define where it falls on the continuum. For example, the drive produced by hunger leads to eating large quantities of food in a short period of time (McHugh & Slavney, 1998). In contrast to orderly behaviors, where the physiological need is followed by satiation once the behavior is emitted, disorderly behavior features abbreviated or absent satiation. For instance, extremely abbreviated satiation is seen with cocaine dependence, where the behavioral sequence is that of drug-seeking, drug attainment, consumption, and recovery from substance use. The consumption and recovery from substance use are very short-lived behaviors that quickly lead to the depletion of both drugs and resources to pay for drugs (McHugh & Slavney, 1998). A disorderly behavior is also one where the behavior is displayed in place of or at the expense of other behaviors. For example, alcohol is used rather than caring for children or attending work.

Rewards as Constructs

Another important concept is the idea of rewards as constructs. Expanding on the definition of construct above, construct can also be defined as a collection of related ideas or behaviors that are associated in a meaningful way. The construct itself cannot be measured directly, but only through measurable indicator variables. Certainly, there are tangible items that tend to be valued by most individuals across many cultures, for example money. However, for an item to be a reward, it must be a desired item, and the value or desire placed on any item varies among individuals and depends upon the person's past experiences, the current situation, and the amount of behavior required to receive the reward. An example of when money may not be a reward is if someone was on a desert island and had no place to spend the money or could not use the money to secure a valued item such as water for survival. Rewards can also be intangible and dynamic. What might be rewarding to someone at one point in time may not later in life function as a reward. For example, a lollipop might function as a reward for a young child but not a teenager.

Motivation as a Construct

As discussed in several of the theories above, motivation is necessary for learning to take place. Motivation for the treatment of substance use disorders is commonly regarded as critical for patients engaging in treatment and ceasing substance use. The construct of motivation has been challenging to define and operationalize, especially given its relationship with "self-control" and "willpower." In past years motivation has been viewed as a trait, but now science is moving to show it is a malleable state. Motivation has been described as multidimensional, dynamic, and modifiable, and as important to help change behavior (Miller & Rollnick, 2002). Motivation has been measured in various ways using diverse methods. Two important constructs of motivation that have received wide attention are treatment readiness and resistance. It is expected that patients with high readiness and low resistance will be most successful in treatment. It has been shown that treatment readiness predicts treatment retention, while treatment resistance predicts substance use (Longshore & Teruya, 2006).

One model that attempts to quantify motivation is the transtheoretical model of change (e.g., Prochaska & DiClemente, 1982). This model describes behavior change as a process that has cycles, and patients can fluidly move back and forth between different stages of motivation. The model has several main constructs, including stages of change, decisional balance, self-efficacy, and processes of change (Prochaska & Velicer, 1997). For the stages-of-change construct, individuals move through five main stages as their behavior changes from having no intention to change to adopting and maintaining behavior change. The model proposes that different interventions are required for individuals at different stages of motivation. Thus, accurate determination of the stage of change is an essential component of the model. There is an ever-growing body of research to both support and refute the efficacy of the stages-of-change model as an essential component in understanding abstinence from substance use, and these conflicting results may be related to the varying methods and tools used to measure and categorize patients into the stages of change (Littell & Girvin, 2002).

Recovery as a Construct

Recovery has been a construct discussed in the field of substance use disorder treatment for many decades. The aspects of recovery that make up the construct include the multiple elements that are part of a healthy lifestyle (e.g., abstinence from substance use, fulfilling relationships with substance-free family and friends, contributing to the maintenance or betterment of society). It has also been a foundational construct for Twelve Step programs such as Alcoholics Anonymous and Narcotics Anonymous (Davidson & White, 2007). Recovery is seen as a nonlinear path, and active ingredients of recovery-oriented systems include both contingency management and Motivational Interviewing (MI) in addition to comprehensive elements of case management services (Davidson & White, 2007) (see Chapter 13 for a discussion of case management with pregnant women).

The Construct of Recovery Applied in Practice

While it is not always provided for patients treated for substance use disorders, there is widespread acceptance that they need long-term management of multiple life aspects to help them make sustained, positive life changes. For pregnant and parenting women, six components of substance use treatment programming, each of which can be considered under the umbrella of recovery, were significantly and positively associated with key substance use treatment outcomes (e.g., treatment completion, length of stay, decreased use of substances, reduced mental health symptoms, improved birth outcomes, employment, self-reported health status, and HIV risk reduction). The six components of care are child care, prenatal care, women-only treatment centers, services and education addressing women-focused topics, mental health services, and comprehensive treatment services (Ashley et al., 2003). Examples of recovery-oriented programs that have published evidence to support their efficacy for treating substance use disorders in pregnant and parenting women include comprehensive care programs like the modified therapeutic community of PROTOTYPES (e.g., Brown et al., 1996). Examples of recovery-oriented programs that provide agonist medication as a part of the complete treatment of opioid-dependent pregnant patients include "Family Center" (Thomas Jefferson University, Philadelphia, PA), a comprehensive outpatient treatment program for pregnant and parenting women; "My Sister's Place," a long-term residential treatment program; "Center for Addiction and Pregnancy" (Johns Hopkins University, Baltimore, MD) which has an assisted living unit and an intensive outpatient treatment program; and the "Horizons" program (University of North Carolina, Chapel Hill, NC), which offers both residential and intensive outpatient treatment.

EXAMPLES OF EVIDENCE-BASED TREATMENTS THAT USE THE ABOVE THEORIES IN THE FOUNDATION OF THEIR APPROACH

Motivational Interviewing and motivational enhancement therapy

MI is a patient-centered approach that helps patients explore ambivalence, how to resolve ambivalence, and how to commit to behavioral change (Miller, 1983). MI evolved from clinical observation as well as Carl Rogers's person-centered counseling approach style (Rogers, 1959), Bem's self-perception theory (e.g., that individuals develop attitudes by observing their own behavior and concluding what attitudes must have caused them; Bem, 1972), and cognitive dissonance (e.g., a motivational drive to reduce dissonance by either changing or justifying their attitudes, beliefs, and behaviors; Festinger, 1957). Thus, the interviewer's goal is to assist the patient in evoking her own "change talk." Change talk includes the patient stating her need, desire, ability, and reasons for behavior change. To facilitate these statements, the provider uses reflective listening and periodic summaries of the patient's own change talk that clarify and amplify her self-motivational statements (Miller & Rollnick, 2002). MI has two distinct phases: increasing motivation for change, and then commitment consolidation (Miller & Rollnick, 2002). The most important element of change talk is the strength of commitment language used—specifically, the pattern of commitment language across the session predicted drug abstinence. Need, desire, ability, and reasons did not predict change, but all four types of change talk did predict the emergence of commitment, and commitment was a prognostic indicator of behavior change. Also, the patient's initial level of motivation in an MI session was unrelated to outcome; instead, the commitment strength during the final minutes of the interview most strongly predicted behavior change (Amrhein et al., 2003).

MI has been found to be effective for reducing substance use (Miller, 1983) in nonpregnant populations. Its largest effects were reported when it was compared to no treatment (Gentilello et al. 1999), a wait-list control (Kelly et al., 2000), or education (Graeber et al., 2003), or, importantly, when it was added to standard treatment (e.g., Brown & Miller, 1993).

Among pregnant women, MI has shown either no effects (Osterman & Dyehouse, 2012) or promising outcomes in reducing alcohol use (Handmaker et al., 1999). MI has not been shown to reduce smoking in low-income (Stotts et al., 2004; Tappin et al., 2005) or methadone-maintained samples (Haug et al., 2004).

In combination with behavioral incentives for drug abstinence and case management provided to pregnant women enrolled in prenatal care but not enrolled in substance use treatment, MI has been shown to improve maternal outcomes of reduced substance use at a rate similar to the rate found for pregnant women given MI and behavioral incentives (Jones et al., 2004). For pregnant women enrolled in prenatal care but not enrolled in substance use treatment, patients who were compliant with four sessions of MI delivered babies with a higher average birth weight than patients who completed zero to three sessions (Jones et al., 2002). Moreover, MI has been successfully used as a part of a comprehensive treatment intervention to reduce substance use and to improve treatment retention and neonatal outcomes of pregnant women with heroin and cocaine dependence compared to participants without such intervention (e.g., Jones et al., 2011). In summary, while MI appears to be a promising approach when provided as a part of a comprehensive treatment package, more research is needed to determine if and how it facilitates behavior changes among individuals who use illicit substances, especially those patients who are pregnant.

Cognitive-Behavioral Intervention Approaches

Cognitive-behavioral intervention approaches are based on the theory that learning processes play a critical role in the development of maladaptive behavioral patterns. People learn to identify and correct problematic behaviors.

Cognitive-behavioral approaches, such as relapse prevention, are grounded in social learning theories and behavioral learning theory principles like operant conditioning. The aspects of these strategies that differentiate them from more traditional recovery models like Alcoholics/Narcotics Anonymous include focusing on a functional analysis of substance use (e.g., understanding substance use as it relates to the antecedents and consequences of substance use) and training patients in skills to support abstinence (e.g., recognize and avoid times or occasions when there is a risk of substance use and learn and apply coping skills if avoidance of these situations is not possible; Carroll, 1998). Cognitive-behavioral strategies have been successfully used in treating alcohol use disorders (see Miller & Wilbourne, 2002, for a review) and substance use disorders such as cocaine abuse (e.g., Carroll et al., 1991).

Several studies have demonstrated that cognitive-behavioral therapy has a "sleeper effect": the effects of treatment are shown long after treatment is over (e.g., Carroll et al., 2000). Despite the emerging empirical support for use of cognitive-behavioral therapy in substance-dependent populations, additional research is needed to address its limitations. Cognitive-behavioral therapy is a comparatively complex approach, and training providers to implement this approach effectively can be challenging. Strategies for addressing these issues include greater emphasis on understanding the mechanisms of action of cognitive-behavioral therapy so that ineffective components can be removed and treatment delivery can be simplified and shortened and perhaps even accomplished by computer or other automated means. Strategies for enhancing acceptance and effective implementation of cognitive-behavioral therapy by the clinical community are also needed (Carroll & Onken, 2005). Importantly, it remains to be determined in which populations of pregnant substance users these cognitive therapies will be most effective.

Neither MI nor cognitive-behavioral strategies have shown high promise for reducing or eliminating cigarette smoking among pregnant women (e.g., Pollak et al., 2007). A pilot study in substance-using pregnant women that used a combination of MI and cognitive-behavioral therapy also showed decreases in substance use by almost 50% from baseline and suggests promising data for a randomized controlled trial with a formal comparison of the intervention to no or usual care (Yonkers et al., 2009). Cognitive-behavioral treatment has also been shown to be effective in reducing HIV injection drug risk behaviors among methadone-maintained pregnant women (O'Neill et al., 1996).

While there is a lack of randomized controlled trials examining the efficacy of cognitive-behavioral treatment for reducing substance use and improving maternal and neonatal outcomes for pregnant women with substance use disorders, numerous programs have been described in the literature that feature, among their many components of comprehensive care, aspects of relapse prevention and other cognitive skills-based training (e.g., Jansson et al., 1996; Kaltenbach et al., 1998; Mosley, 1996).While these comprehensive care programs have never been tested in a dismantling study to determine their active ingredients, it is an almost universal belief that these cognitive-behavioral components help to establish and maintain abstinence.

Contingency Management

One of the most important scientific advances in the treatment of substance use disorders was the discovery that the behaviors making up these disorders follow the laws of learning and conditioning (see Bigelow & Silverman, 1999, for a review). Both preclinical and clinical literature have repeatedly shown that substance use is a form of operant behavior that is sensitive to environmental consequences (e.g., Cosgrove & Carroll, 2003; Higgins et al., 1994a,b, 2000). Therefore, substance-use–related behaviors can be altered when the environment is arranged in ways that makes substance use less attractive.

Contingency management treatments take advantage of the power of alternative positive reinforcers to make abstinence a more immediately attractive option than substance use and to shape behavioral choices toward sustained abstinence. Contingency management is characterized by the systematic delivery of or withholding of reinforcing or punishing consequences that depend on the presence or absence, respectively, of the target response (Higgins & Petry, 1999).

Specific elements that are considered the "active ingredients" of contingency management include identification of a clinically relevant target behavior, an objective measure of that behavior that is performed frequently, patient and provider negotiation and agreement on the selection of a desired reinforcer, a consistent and immediate temporal link between the target behavior, and delivery of the desired reinforcer (Fig. 2.1).

Finally, contingency management was conceived as a method for enhancing treatment in the presence of other therapeutic intervention(s), not as a sole or primary intervention approach.

Contingency management has been utilized to promote a multitude of healthy behaviors in patients with substance use disorders. Examples include reducing cigarette smoking (Dunn et al., 2008); increasing adherence to naltrexone therapy (e.g., Preston et al., 1999) and antiretroviral therapy (e.g., Rigsby et al., 2000); and improving attendance (Silverman et al., 2001) and increasing productivity (Wong et al., 2004) at vocational training in methadone-maintenance patients.

- Identification of a clinically relevant target behavior (e.g., drug abstinence),
- Objective measurement of the behavior (e.g., urine tests revealing recent drug use or abstinence)
- Performing the measurement frequently (e.g., no less than once a week),
- With the patient, selecting a desired reinforcer (e.g., goods and services with monetary value),
- Consistent and immediate temporal link between the target behavior (submission of a urine sample that tests negative for drugs of abuse) and delivery of the desired reinforcer (e.g., gift certificate to a grocery store that the patient likes to visit).

Figure 2.1 Examples of Active Ingredients of Specific Elements of Contingency Management

For pregnant women, contingency management has been successfully used to promote cessation from cigarette smoking (e.g., Heil et al., 2008), increase cocaine abstinence rates (Elk et al., 1995; Elk et al., 1998), and increase treatment attendance and abstinence from concomitant substances compared to a non-incentive schedule (Jones et al., 2001).

Most recently, scientific attention has focused on examining the efficacy of contingency management for promoting healthy behaviors in patients with substance use disorders during pregnancy. For example, a recently completed study assessing the effectiveness of contingency management for reducing prenatal tobacco use found that cigarette smoking may be reduced significantly among methadone-maintained pregnant women with the use of 12 weeks of contingent reinforcement for gradual reductions in breath carbon monoxide levels (Tuten et al., 2012).

Community Reinforcement Approach

Originally developed for use with individuals with alcohol use disorders, the community reinforcement approach (CRA) is based on the theory that substance use is maintained by substance-associated reinforcers and the absence of non–substance-related reinforcers. Thus, like contingency management, CRA is based on behavioral learning theory (Smith et al., 2001). CRA focuses on building a substance-free lifestyle by fostering rewarding activities in the areas of employment, recreation, and socializing that can provide alternative reinforcers over the long term. The intervention approach of CRA is based upon the cognitive learning theory and delivers traditional relapse-prevention skills building (e.g., drug refusal, assertiveness training), emphasizing explicit goal setting and outreach efforts designed to remove barriers and ensure goal attainment (e.g., Abbott et al., 1998).

Inpatient, outpatient, and homeless CRA participants all show less alcohol use than control participants (Azrin, 1976; Azrin et al., 1982; Hunt & Azrin, 1973; Smith et al., 1998). These results with CRA have been replicated in a large-scale study (Miller et al., 2001). CRA has also been successfully used with methadone-maintained individuals (Bickel et al., 1987) as well as adapted for use with cocaine-dependent patients (e.g., Higgins et al., 1991, 1993, 1994a,b) to reduce substance use.

CRA has also been adapted for use with non–substance-using significant others of substance-using patients considered to be treatment-resistant (Kirby et al., 1999; Meyers et al., 2003; Miller et al., 1999). In these studies adaptations of CRA included education about substance use disorders, positive consequences of alcohol abstinence, and healthy recreational and social activities that can be done as couples. While several CRA manuals have been published (e.g., for cocaine treatment, see Budney & Higgins, 1998; for alcohol treatment, see Meyers & Smith, 1995), the specific content of CRA varies depending on the clinical population and individual patient needs, but it usually has several key components (Fig. 2.2).

Many of the studies examining the efficacy of CRA to treat substance use disorders used CRA in combination with contingency management. This combination showed better treatment outcomes (e.g., drug abstinence, treatment retention) than more standard counseling for substance use or CRA without contingency management (Bickel et al. 1997; Higgins et al. 1991, 1993, 1994b, 2003; Jones et al., 2005). The only CRA + contingency management trial that isolated the contribution of CRA to improved substance use treatment outcome showed that CRA with contingency management increased treatment retention, cocaine abstinence, and reduced alcohol use compared to contingency management without CRA (Higgins et al., 2003).

For pregnant women, the only known trial examining CRA is a trial funded by the National Institute on Drug Abuse with preliminary results suggesting

- Address major barriers to treatment engagement in the first few CRA sessions
- Provide vocational counseling (e.g., Job Club, see Azrin & Besalel-Azrin, 1980) for unemployed patients
- Use functional analysis of substance use to understand the antecedents and consequences of the behavior
- Provide behavioral therapy for couples as needed, for patients who have a partner who is either in need of substance use treatment or who is already drug-free
- Cognitive behavioral skills training is given to address abstinence initiation or relapse risk (e.g., drug refusal, social skills, and mood management training).
- If available, monitored medication therapy is offered for substance use use (e.g., Antabuse for alcohol problems or methadone for opioid dependence).

Figure 2.2 Examples of Key Ingredients of a Community Reinforcement Approach (CRA)

that, compared to usual substance use treatment, CRA plus contingency management and MI given to pregnant patients with substance use disorders produces greater treatment utilization and improved abstinence from substance use, with shorter hospital stays for the neonate (Jones et al., 2011).

SUMMARY

This chapter has demonstrated that many of the interventions used to treat women with substance use disorders during pregnancy are based on combinations of behavioral, cognitive, and social learning theories. Contingency management has the greatest depth and breath of empirical data to support its use in changing substance use behaviors of pregnant patients. Moreover, the majority of the empirical evidence regarding the efficacy of treatments for substance use disorders during pregnancy shows that combinations of treatments are most successful. However, it is important to explicitly identify the theoretical foundation of the treatment(s). It is possible to use different theories in treatment successfully if the providers ensure that there is a unified philosophy of the treatment approach.

REFERENCES

Abbott, P. J., Weller, S. B., Delaney, H. D., & Moore, B. A. (1998). Community reinforcement approach in the treatment of opiate addicts. *American Journal of Drug Alcohol Abuse, 24*, 17–30.

Amrhein, P. C., Miller, W. R., Yahne, C. E., Palmer, M., & Fulcher, L. (2003). Client commitment language during motivational interviewing predicts drug use outcomes. *Journal of Consulting and Clinical Psychology, 71*, 862–878.

Ashley, O. S., Marsden, M. E., & Brady, T. M. (2003). Effectiveness of substance abuse treatment programming for women: A review. *American Journal of Drug and Alcohol Abuse, 29*, 19–53.

Azrin, N. H. (1976). Improvements in the community-reinforcement approach to alcoholism. *Behavior Research and Therapy, 14*(5), 339–348.

Azrin, N. H. & Besalel-Azrin, V. A. (1980). *Job club counselor's manual: A behavioral approach to vocational counseling.* Baltimore: University Park Press.

Azrin, N. H., Sisson, R. W., Meyers, R., & Godley, M. (1982). Alcoholism treatment by disulfiram and community reinforcement therapy. *Journal of Behavior Therapy and Experimental Psychiatry, 13*(2), 105–112.

Bem, D. J. (1972). Self-perception theory. In L. Berkowitz (Ed.), *Advances in experimental social psychology* (Vol. 6, pp. 1–62). New York: Academic Press.

Bickel, W. K., Amass, L., Higgins, S. T., Badger, G. J., & Esch, R. A. (1997). Effects of adding behavioral treatment to opiod detoxification with buprenorphine. *Journal of Consulting and Clinical Psychology, 65*(5), 803–810.

Bickel, W. K., Marion, I., & Lowinson, J. H. (1987). The treatment of alcoholic methadone patients: a review. *Journal of Substance Abuse Treatment, 4*(1), 15–19.

Bigelow, G. E., & Silverman, K. (1999). Theoretical and empirical foundations of contingency management treatments for drug abuse. In S. T. Higgins & K. Silverman (Eds.), *Motivating behavior change among illicit-drug abusers: Research on contingency management interventions* (pp. 15–31). Washington, DC: American Psychological Association.

Brown, J. M., & Miller, W. R. (1993). Impact of motivational interviewing on participation and outcome in residential alcoholism treatment. *Psychology of Addictive Behaviors, 7*, 211.

Brown, V. B., Sanchez, S., Zweben, J. E., & Aly, T. (1996). Challenges in moving from a traditional therapeutic community to a women and children's TC model. *Journal of Psychoactive Drugs, 28*(1), 39–46.

Budney, A. J., & Higgins, S. T. (1998). *Treating cocaine addiction: A community reinforcement plus vouchers approach.* Rockville, MD: NIDA.

Carroll K. A. (1998). *Cognitive-Behavioral Approach: Treating Cocaine Addiction.* National Institute on Drug Abuse. NIH Publication Number 98–4308.

Carroll, K. M., Nich, C., Ball, S. A., McCance, E., Frankforter, T. L., & Rounsaville, B. J. (2000). One-year follow-up of disulfiram and psychotherapy for cocaine-alcohol users: sustained effects of treatment. *Addiction, 95*(9), 1335–1349.

Carroll, K. M., & Onken, L. S. (2005). Behavioral therapies for drug abuse. *American Journal of Psychiatry, 162*(8), 1452–1460.

Carroll, K. M., Rounsaville, B. J., & Keller, D. S. (1991). Relapse prevention strategies for the treatment of cocaine abuse. *American Journal of Drug and Alcohol Abuse, 17*(3), 249–265.

Cosgrove, K. P., & Carroll, M. E. (2003). Effects of a non-drug reinforcer, saccharin, on oral self-administration of phencyclidine in male and female rhesus monkeys. *Psychopharmacology (Berl), 170*(1), 9–16.

Davidson, L., & White, W. (2007). The concept of recovery as an organizing principle for integrating mental health and addiction services. *Journal of Behavior Health Service and Research, 34*(2), 109–120.

Dunn, K. E., Sigmon, S. C., Thomas, C. S., Heil, S. H., & Higgins, S. T. (2008). Voucher-based contingent reinforcement of smoking abstinence among methadone-maintained patients: a pilot study. *Journal of Applied Behavioral Analysis, 41*(4), 527–538.

Elk, R., Mangus, L., Rhoades, H., Andres, R., & Grabowski, J. (1998). Cessation of cocaine use during pregnancy: effects of contingency management interventions on maintaining abstinence and complying with prenatal care. *Addictive Behaviors, 23*(1), 57–64.

Elk, R., Schmitz, J., Spiga, R., Rhoades, H., Andres, R., & Grabowski, J. (1995). Behavioral treatment of cocaine-dependent pregnant women and TB-exposed patients. *Addictive Behaviors, 20*(4), 533–542.

Festinger, L. (1957). *A theory of cognitive dissonance.* Evanston, IL: Row, Peterson.

Gentilello, L. M., Rivara, F. P., Donovan, D. M., Jurkovich, G. J., Daranciang, E., Dunn, C. W., Villaveces, A., Copass, M., & Ries, R. R. (1999). Alcohol interventions in a trauma center as a means of reducing the risk of injury recurrence. *Annals of Surgery, 230*(4), 473–483.

Graeber, D. A., Moyers, T. B., Griffith, G., Guajardo, E., & Tonigan, S. (2003). A pilot study comparing motivational interviewing and an educational intervention in patients with schizophrenia and alcohol use disorders. *Community Mental Health Journal, 39,* 189–202.

Gross, R. D. (1992). *Psychology: the science of mind and behaviour* (2nd ed.). London: Hodder & Stoughton.

Handmaker, N. S., Miller, W. R., & Manicke, M. (1999). Findings of a pilot study of motivational interviewing with pregnant drinkers. *Journal of Studies on Alcohol and Drugs, 60*(2), 285–287.

Haug, N. A., Svikis, D. S., & Diclemente, C. (2004). Motivational enhancement therapy for nicotine dependence in methadone-maintained pregnant women. *Psychology of Addictive Behaviors, 18*(3), 289–292.

Heil, S. H., Higgins, S. T., Bernstein, I. M., Solomon, L. J., Rogers, R. E., Thomas, C. S., Badger, G. J., & Lynch, M. E. (2008). Effects of voucher-based incentives on abstinence from cigarette smoking and fetal growth among pregnant women. *Addiction, 103*(6), 1009–1018.

Higgins, S. T., Bickel, W. K., & Hughes, J. R. (1994a). Influence of an alternative reinforcer on human cocaine self-administration. *Life Science, 55,* 179–187.

Higgins, S. T., Budney, A. J., Bickel, W. K., Foerg, F. E., Donham, R., & Badger, G. J. (1994b). Incentives improve outcome in outpatient behavioral treatment of cocaine dependence. *Archives of General Psychiatry,51*(7), 568–576.

Higgins, S. T., Budney, A. J., Bickel, W. K., Hughes, J. R., Foerg, F., & Badger, G. (1993). Achieving cocaine abstinence with a behavioral approach. *American Journal of Psychiatry, 150*(5), 763–769.

Higgins, S. T., Delaney, D. D., Budney, A. J., Bickel, W. K., Hughes, J. R., Foerg, F., & Fenwick, J. W. (1991). A behavioral approach to achieving initial cocaine abstinence. *American Journal of Psychiatry, 148*(9), 1218–1224.

Higgins, S. T., & Petry, N. M. (1999). Contingency management: incentives for sobriety. *Alcohol Research & Health, 23*(2), 121–127.

Higgins, S. T., Sigmon, S. C., Wong, C. J., Heil, S. H., Badger, G. J., Donham, R., Dantona, R. L., & Anthony, S. (2003). Community reinforcement therapy for cocaine-dependent outpatients. *Archives of General Psychiatry, 60,* 1043–1052.

Hunt, G. M., & Azrin, N. H. (1973). A community-reinforcement approach to alcoholism. *Behaviour Research and Therapy, 11*(1), 91–104.

Jansson, L. M., Svikis, D., Lee, J., Paluzzi, P., Rutigliano, P., & Hackerman F. (1996). Pregnancy and addiction. A comprehensive care model. *Journal of Substance Abuse Treatment, 13*(4), 321–329.

Jones, H. E., Haug, N., Silverman, K., Stitzer, M., & Svikis, D. (2001). The effectiveness of incentives in enhancing treatment attendance and drug abstinence in methadone-maintained pregnant women. *Drug and Alcohol Dependence, 61*(3), 297–306.

Jones, H. E., O'Grady, K. E., & Tuten, M. (2011). Reinforcement-based treatment improves the maternal treatment and neonatal outcomes of pregnant patients enrolled in comprehensive care treatment. *American Journal on Addictions, 20*(3), 196–204.

Jones, H. E., Svikis, D., Rosado, J., Tuten, M., & Kulstad, J. L. (2004). What if they do not want treatment? Lessons learned from intervention studies of non-treatment-seeking, drug-using pregnant women. *American Journal on Addictions, 13*(4), 342–357.

Jones, H. E., Svikis, D. S., & Tran, G. (2002). Patient compliance and maternal/infant outcomes in pregnant drug-using women. *Substance Use and Misuse, 37*(11), 1411–1222.

Jones, H. E., Wong, C. J., Tuten, M., & Stitzer, M. L. (2005). Reinforcement-based therapy: 12-month evaluation of an outpatient drug-free treatment for heroin abusers. *Drug and Alcohol Dependence, 79*(2), 119–128.

Kaltenbach, K., Berghella, V., & Finnegan, L. (1998). Opioid dependence during pregnancy: Effects and management. *Obstetrical and Gynecological Clinics of North America, 25*(1), 139–151.

Kelly, A. B., Halford, W. K., & Young, R. M. (2000). Maritally distressed women with alcohol problems: the impact of a short-term alcohol-focused intervention on drinking behaviour and marital satisfaction. *Addiction, 95*(10), 1537–1549.

Kirby, K. C., Marlowe, D. B., Festinger, D. S., Garvey, K. A., & La Monaca, V. (1999). Community reinforcement training for family and significant others of drug abusers: a unilateral intervention to increase treatment entry of drug users. *Drug and Alcohol Dependence, 56*(1), 85–96.

Littell, J. H., & Girvin, H. (2002). Stages of change: A critique. *Behavior Modification, 26*(2), 223–273.

Longshore, D., & Teruya, C. (2006). Treatment motivation in drug users: a theory-based analysis. *Drug and Alcohol Dependence, 81*(2), 179–188.

McHugh, P. R., & Slavney, P. R. (1998). *The perspectives of psychiatry*. Baltimore: Johns Hopkins University Press.

Meyers, R., & Smith, J.E. (1995). *A clinical guide to alcohol treatment. The community reinforcement approach*. New York: Guilford Press.

Meyers, R. J., Smith, J. E., & Lash, D. N. (2003). The community reinforcement approach. *Recent Developments in Alcoholism, 16*, 183–195.

Miller, N. E., & Dollard, J. (1941). *Social learning and imitation*. New Haven, CT: Yale University Press.

Miller, W. R. (1983). Motivational Interviewing with problem drinkers. *Behavioral Psychotherapy, 11*, 147–172.

Miller, W. R., Meyers, R. J., & Hiller-Sturmhöfel, S. (1999). The community-reinforcement approach. *Alcohol Research & Health, 23*(2), 116–121.

Miller, W. R., Meyers, R. J., Tonigan, J. S., & Grant, K. A. (2001). Community reinforcement and traditional approaches: findings of a controlled trial. *Addictions, 9*, 79–86.

Miller, W. R., & Rollnick, S. (2002). *Motivational interviewing: Preparing people for change*. New York: Guilford Press.

Miller, W. R., & Wilbourne, P. L. (2002). Mesa Grande: a methodological analysis of clinical trials of treatments for alcohol use disorders. *Addiction, 97*(3), 265–277.

Mosley, T. M. (1996). PROTOTYPES: an urban model program of treatment and recovery services for dually diagnosed perinatal program participants. *Journal of Psychoactive Drugs, 28*(4), 381–388.

O'Neill, K., Baker, A., Cooke, M., Collins, E., Heather, N., & Wodak, A. (1996). Evaluation of a cognitive-behavioural intervention for pregnant injecting drug users at risk of HIV infection. *Addiction, 91*(8), 1115–1125.

Ormrod, J. E. (1999). *Human learning* (3rd ed.). Upper Saddle River, NJ: Prentice-Hall.

Osterman, R. L., & Dyehouse, J. (2012). Effects of a motivational interviewing intervention to decrease prenatal alcohol use. *Western Journal of Nursing Research, 34*(4),434–454.

Pollak, K. I., Oncken, C. A., Lipkus, I. M., Lyna, P., Swamy, G. K., Pletsch, P. K., Peterson, B. L., Heine, R. P., Brouwer, R. J., Fish, L., & Myers, E. R. (2007). Nicotine replacement and behavioral therapy for smoking cessation in pregnancy. *American Journal of Preventive Medicine, 33*(4), 297–305.

Preston, K. L., Silverman, K., Umbricht, A., DeJesus, A., Montoya, I. D., & Schuster, C. R. (1999). Improvement in naltrexone treatment compliance with contingency management. *Drug and Alcohol Dependence, 54*(2), 127–135.

Prochaska, J. O., & DiClemente, C. C. (1982). Trans-theoretical therapy—toward a more integrative model of change. *Psychotherapy: Theory, Research and Practice, 19*(3), 276–288.

Prochaska, J. O., & Velicer, W. F. (1997). The transtheoretical model of health behavior change. *American Journal of Health Promotion, 12*, 38–48.

Rigsby, M. O., Rosen, M. I., Beauvais, J. E., Cramer, J. A., Rainey, P. M., O'Malley, S. S., Dieckhaus, K. D., & Rounsaville, B. J. (2000). Cue-dose training with monetary reinforcement: pilot study of an antiretroviral adherence intervention. *Journal of General Internal Medicine, 15*(12), 841–847.

Rogers, C. (1959). A theory of therapy, personality and interpersonal relationships as developed in the client-centered framework. In S. Koch (Ed.), *Psychology: A study of a science. Vol. 3: Formulations of the person and the social context* (pp. 184–256). New York: McGraw Hill.

Rotter, J. B. (1982). *The development and applications of social learning theory.* New York: Praeger.

Silverman, K., Svikis, D., Robles, E., Stitzer, M. L.,& Bigelow, G. E. (2001). A reinforcement-based therapeutic workplace for the treatment of drug abuse: six-month abstinence outcomes. *Experimental and Clinical Psychopharmacology, 9*(1), 14–23.

Skinner, B. F. (1971). *Beyond freedom and dignity.* Indianapolis, IN: Hackett Publishing Company, Inc.

Smith, J. E., Meyers, R. J., & Delaney, H. D. (1998). The community reinforcement approach with homeless alcohol-dependent individuals. *Journal of Consulting and Clinical Psychology, 66*(3), 541–548.

Smith, J. E., Meyers, R. J., & Miller, W. R. (2001). The community reinforcement approach to the treatment of substance use disorders. *American Journal on Addictions, 10*, 51–59.

Stotts, A. L., DeLaune, K. A., Schmitz, J. M., & Grabowski, J. (2004). Impact of a motivational intervention on mechanisms of change in low-income pregnant smokers. *Addictive Behaviors, 29*(8), 1649–1657.

Tappin, D. M., Lumsden, M. A., Gilmour, W. H., Crawford, F., McIntyre, D., Stone, D. H., Webber, R., MacIndoe, S., & Mohammed, E. (2005). Randomized controlled trial of home based motivational interviewing by midwives to help pregnant smokers quit or cut down. *British Medical Journal, 331*, 373–377.

Tuten, M., Fitzsimons, H., Chisolm, M. S., Nuzzo, P. A., & Jones, H. E. (2012). Contingent incentives reduce cigarette smoking among pregnant, methadone-maintained women: Results of an initial feasibility and efficacy randomized clinical trial. *Addiction, 107(10),1868–1877.*

Wong, C. J., Dillon, E. M., Sylvest, C., & Silverman, K. (2004). Evaluation of a modified contingency management intervention for consistent attendance in therapeutic workplace participants. *Drug and Alcohol Dependence, 74*(3), 319–323.

Yonkers, K. A., Howell, H. B., Allen, A. E., Ball, S. A., Pantalon, M. V., Rounsaville, B. J. (2009). A treatment for substance abusing pregnant women. *Archives of Womens Mental Health, 12*(4), 221–227.

3

Why Is Treatment Context Important?

OVERVIEW

This chapter builds upon the previous chapter on the theoretical basis for treating women with substance use disorders while pregnant. The previous chapter provided two overall conclusions. First, using treatments based upon social learning theory such as cognitive-behavioral treatments plus contingency management is a powerful way of engaging, retaining, and promoting drug abstinence and other associated positive life behaviors in patients receiving treatment for substance use disorders. Second, comprehensive programs that treat substance use disorders in pregnant women use eclectic approaches and many of these approaches have a foundation in social learning theory.

In this chapter we review the factors that provide a healthy atmosphere of reinforcement so that patients have a respectful, supported, and affirming treatment experience. These types of activities are consistent with a recovery-oriented model of care. The recovery-oriented model of care is also used in a family-centered approach to behavioral health in a general medical care context. In this chapter we provide practical ways to review, develop, and maintain a high degree of patient-focused care in a program treating substance use disorders in pregnant women. Finally, we summarize the key points from the discussion of the importance of treatment context.

INTRODUCTION

Patients who are treated for substance use disorders deserve to receive the best possible treatment. The clinical and support staff providing these life-saving services should have the expectation that their work will be performed in a nurturing, supportive, and positive environment. As discussed in Chapter 2, rewards may have an important role in both bringing about and sustaining behavior change on the part of the patient; however, for these rewards to have their full effect, they must be given and received in a treatment setting that is supportive, nurturing, and affirming of its patients. To create a healthy atmosphere of reinforcement, treatment for substance use disorders must be provided in a setting where the physical environment conveys care and respect, and where every staff interaction, from the front-desk receptionist to the program director, is viewed as an opportunity for a therapeutic contact. The language used to talk with patients and between patients must convey respect, understanding, and messages of optimism for positive behavioral change in all patients, regardless of their current or past histories with treatment.

KEYS TO ENSURING AND MAINTAINING A HEALTHY ATMOSPHERE OF REINFORCEMENT

The often-unspoken reality of any type of health care, including substance use disorder treatment services, is that these services are a business. Explicitly acknowledging this fact does not negate the value of the therapeutic relationship; in fact, it can serve as an important reminder of the value of the patient to the clinic employees and administration. Patient-oriented and family-oriented service and effective therapy share the same basic essence: forming a relationship with customers. This relationship must be one that the individual customer—in this case a patient—feels that she would like to establish and maintain.

One focus of treatment is encouraging the patient to form and maintain close positive relationships with drug-free others. Many pregnant women with substance use disorders have limited positive role models for developing these healthy relationships. This lack of experience with rewarding interpersonal relationships can also be seen in their relationships with clinic and staff members. While what the provider says is important, patients will largely judge the provider by his or her actions and tone, which serve as the underlying theme of patient-oriented care.

The following keys are adapted from three consumer-oriented sources (Ahire, 2007; Tahir, 2012; Ward, 2008). Their use will help maximize treatment entry, engagement, and retention.

Be Available

Being available to patients is conveyed in many ways, from always answering the phone, to having convenient clinic hours, to having an emergency hotline number. Each phone number that is given to a potential or active patient should have either call forwarding or an answering service. As often as possible, a "real person" should answer the phone when it rings. Patients like talking to people, not automated machines. It is also important to emphasize, monitor, and reward professional phone etiquette by the providers and clinic staff (Fig. 3.1).

The clinic's hours should be convenient for patients. For example, being open only in the morning may pose challenges for patients who have long commutes or who work night shifts. Having the clinic open in the early evening may help working patients use treatment services while still maintaining gainful employment. The clinic's hours should also take into account the schedule of the public transportation system, if one is available.

Having weekend hours to provide treatment on high-risk days that can be triggers for patients can convey an understanding of the dependence process and the ability of the treatment facility to meet patients' needs.

---

1. *Answer* all incoming phone calls quickly (by the third or fourth ring).
2. *Have a script for answering the phone.* For example, the person answering the phone should say "Hello. You have reached the [Insert name] Treatment Clinic and I am [insert name of the staff member]. How may I help you today?" Often the voice at the end of the telephone line is the first or only impression of your clinic a caller will receive.
3. *How you say things matters.* Enunciate clearly, keep your voice volume moderate, and speak slowly and clearly. While in most cases you should be avoid slang or jargon, when used purposefully it can help a patient feel more comfortable and understood.
4. *Convey both empathy and a positive attitude.* Everyone answering the phone should use a voice and vocabulary that conveys care, respect, and a positive attitude. Treat everyone as if you are answering a phone call from a Very Important Person (VIP).
5. *Return all calls within one business day.* This conveys to the caller that she is important and reinforces a favorable impression of the clinic.
6. *Always ask if it's all right to put the caller on hold.* Do not leave people on hold. Offer them choices if possible, such as "That line is still busy. Will you continue to hold or should I have _____ call you back?"
7. *Make sure answering-machine messages are accurate and updated as needed.* For example, if the clinic is closing for a holiday, the message should say so and should also say when the clinic will reopen. Make sure there is a separate message for evenings, nights, and weekends. The message should tell the caller what to do in the case of an emergency (e.g., call 911).
8. *Check on how the clinic's phones are being answered.* Call in and see if the phone is being answered in a professional manner. Reward those individuals who are doing well. Provide regular feedback and booster training on aspects of phone communication.

Figure 3.1 Tips for Excellent Phone Service

Availability also includes the length of time it takes from when the patient enters treatment to when she is seen by the clinic staff person responsible for coordinating her care (e.g., counselor, social worker). This coordinating staff member should meet the patient as soon as possible; if time is limited, this first contact can be brief. This meeting is the patient's first impression of treatment. Some patients view it as the start of their treatment, so it can set the tone for how treatment will be perceived by the patient.

Keep Your Promises

Only make promises that will be kept. Reliability is one of the most important keys to any good relationship. In substance use treatment, where patients often have chaotic lives and little structure or ability to depend on anyone, reliability is vital to maximizing a patient's treatment success. If you say that the patient's appointment will be on Friday at 4 p.m., then you must be there on time to meet with the patient. Think before you give any promise, because when a staff member is not consistent in his or her behavior, there is little chance that the pregnant patient will be likely to establish or maintain her own reliable behavior with regard to treatment. The importance of keeping promises can be critical in matters small or large. For example, if you promise to call a social service worker on behalf of the patient or to bring in a book for her to read, you must keep your word, even if it seems a trivial or offhand commitment to the patient. Not following through on these small and seemingly inconsequential promises can slowly erode the therapeutic relationship (Fig. 3.2).

In summary, be consistent in your behaviors at all times. The therapeutic relationship is a fragile one and can be undermined by what might seem to clinic staff as seemingly minor acts of unreliability—as well as more significant breeches of confidentiality, as discussed in Chapter 1.

Examples of potentially damaging acts include:
- Being late to or missing appointments
- Failing to follow up on something you promised in the last session
- Applying rules inconsistently (e.g., excusing lateness to sessions sometimes but not others)

Figure 3.2 The Value of Consistent Provider Behavior

Listen to Your Patients

Often providers overestimate the amount of real listening that their patients experience. Real listening is conveyed in verbal and nonverbal ways. In Western cultures, eye contact, mirroring the body positioning of the patient, and leaning in, with arms and legs uncrossed, are all nonverbal ways of joining with your patient in listening. Ensuring that there is not physical barrier, like a desk, in between the patient and provider is another aspect of joining with patients. Actively listening to a patient can be conveyed by summarizing for the patient what has been said. As discussed in Chapter 2, Motivational Interviewing is an effective method to teach and refine active listening skills. In substance use disorder treatment, active listening does not usually mean solving the problem for the patient but rather helping to point out to the patient that she has the tools and ability within herself to find the answers to her problems.

Keep the Patient Informed

Providing regular updates about the process and progress of the patient's treatment is important. Patients should be informed of any changes to the treatment regimen, schedule, or programming well in advance of their implementation. The appropriate clinic staff should prepare the patient for the impending changes and repeat information about the change on several occasions. Asking on several occasions if the patient has any concerns or fears about the changes and working with the patient to discuss and appropriately address these concerns will help minimize the opportunities for unpleasant patient interactions. Changes in treatment that affect all patients should be discussed with each patient and reinforced with written postings throughout the clinic and on the clinic website. Posting information without discussing it is an insufficient way to convey changes to patients.

Address Complaints

Listening to complaints can be difficult and unpleasant. Many of us who work with difficult patients on a daily basis have developed self-protective reflexes to respond with skepticism to most patients' complaints. Many times this skepticism is well founded—but giving the complaint appropriate attention will help the patient feel heard and empowered even if she does not like the agency's response to the complaint.

Be Helpful—Even If There's No Immediate Payoff

Often our former patients stop by our clinic to ask for a resource list of housing or other services, to use the phone, to use the computer to look for jobs or other social resources, to use the bathroom, etc. Greeting each past patient and assisting her, within appropriate therapeutic boundaries, can provide a valuable source of positive word-of-mouth "advertising." Women enrolled in a pregnancy and substance use treatment program can feel that they are "kicked to the curb" shortly after delivery. Providing safe boundaries and consistent rules for accessing resources in the clinic can help attract future patients—and maintain the health and well-being of former patients.

Train All Providers, Staff, and Administrators to be Always Helpful, Courteous, and Knowledgeable

Incorporate regular discussions in staff meetings about what is (and isn't) good patient service. Develop regular meetings where staff, providers, and administrators who provide good patient service are publicly rewarded. Include a section on annual evaluations that provides feedback on this aspect of job performance. Most importantly, give all members of the clinic staff enough information and power so that they can provide helpful treatment experiences. Using a "secret shopper/mystery patient" model where all clinic providers, staff, and administrators are unaware of when this will occur and are aware they will be evaluated and given feedback on their interaction with this pseudo-patient will go a long way to promoting a clinic atmosphere that is reinforcing to patients.

Take the Extra Step

Nothing conveys respect and value to a person more than when you make an extra effort. For example, make sure the front-desk receptionist knows each patient by her first name and greets her each day. Providing patients with water, decaffeinated coffee and teas, and light snacks during the day also demonstrates caring and nurturing. Never underestimate the value of small things, as they can be greatly appreciated. An example of a small but powerful reward is having a specific time each week when patients are awarded printed certificates that provide a written summary of the achievement of therapeutic goals. These certificates could be awarded by the therapist in front of the entire patient group. The awarding of the certificate could then be followed by group applause and well wishes.

Maintain a Positive Attitude

The surest way to aggravate an already disagreeable patient is if the provider or staff conveys a negative attitude. Negative attitudes can be conveyed in verbal and nonverbal ways. For example, looking bored, agitated, or irritated will do little to foster a positive interaction with a patient. Accurate empathy is one of the most critical aspects of a therapeutic relationship (e.g., Najavits & Weiss, 1994).

Be Patient

Some patients are easier to work with than others. Some patients may not understand the point the provider is trying to make. For example, many providers who have been in the field for a long time may use a lot of treatment "jargon," and it is easy to forget that patients may not understand the message. Another reason to avoid technical language is that the patient may become frustrated and confused in the face of communications that she fails to understand; in this situation, the provider will miss the opportunity to provide a therapeutic interaction for the patient. Being patient with someone who is frustrated or confused is paramount to effective interaction and treatment response.

Regularly Review the Clinic's Physical Environment

As stated in the opening of this chapter, the clinic's physical environment must convey care and respect, so the inside and outside environment needs to be evaluated regularly. How might it be improved to meet the treatment needs of the patients?

ACCESS TO THE CLINIC
Clear signage can reduce frustration in patients attempting to find the clinic for the first time. The clinic should be well marked and maps and directions of how to get to the clinic should be available on the clinic website and provided to patients before they arrive. The clinic website should include hours of operation, maps and directions, available public transportation, clinic rules, and other such appropriate information.

THE EXTERIOR OF THE CLINIC
How well the exterior of the building is maintained conveys an initial message to patients and their families as to how important, respected, and valued they are. A clean, freshly painted, well-manicured building that is free of trash (including

cigarette butts) and graffiti is part of the initial message sent to the patient about how serious and professional the treatment is that she will receive.

The outside of the clinic and the ability to get to and from the clinic easily are important factors for facilitating treatment entry and attendance. Parking for patients and staff should be provided close to the clinic; if possible, parking for staff and patients should be separate to minimize after-hours communication and interaction. There should be security measures in place such as lighting, surveillance cameras, and security staff (Bailes & Lowery, 2006). Women with substance use disorders may be involved with partners who are abusive, so providing an environment where there are no hidden alleys or places where attackers may hide is important. It should also be the policy that partners, friends, and family may enter the clinic building only if prior arrangements with the clinic have been made.

INTERIOR OF THE CLINIC

Both the outside and inside of the clinic should be aesthetically pleasing and should ensure the safety of patients and staff. Obviously, building codes should be followed allowing for the mobility of physically impaired patients. This rule is especially important for pregnant women, who may be on bed rest or confined to wheelchairs to reduce the risk of premature labor. Security mirrors should be installed to minimize blind spots in the clinic and to allow staff to monitor activity.

The clinic's reception area is the second part of the initial impression. Plants add warmth and a nurturing feel. Make sure the waiting room is stocked with recent magazines and pamphlets on pregnancy, childbirth, and parenting; physical, emotional, and mental health; sexually transmitted diseases; and community resources. Providing both male and female condoms in the reception room and bathroom allows patients free and easy access to an important method for HIV-risk reduction. Instructions for using these condoms are important for proper use. Bulletin boards should be tidy and updated regularly to convey professionalism and concern for patients (Bailes & Lowery, 2006). Even the pictures or inspirational messages that hang on the walls should provide clear messages to patients about hope and optimism. For example, a picture that says "Don't let the turkeys get you down" conveys a very different message than "What you dream you can achieve." Having a phone near the reception desk with a phone book and community resource guides also gives patients tools to help proactively take care of psychosocial service issues. The reception desk should always be staffed, and the staff person should welcome each patient with a friendly greeting.

Often pregnant women in substance use disorder treatment have other children, so having a secure play area for children with several washable classic toys designed for children less than 3 years of age will reduce child-management problems. For example, providing picture books, blocks, soft cars, and/or a pretend kitchen set can keep children occupied. These items need to be regularly disinfected and inspected for safety.

The group counseling rooms should be designed to facilitate therapeutic conversation and safety. Ideally, they should be located away from the common waiting area to protect patient confidentiality. They should be equipped with panic buttons in case of emergency. Group rooms should have comfortable, sturdy chairs that can be easily cleaned. Each room should have a whiteboard or flip chart and materials for writing goals or thoughts for the day, and/or outlining treatment process or goals. Having a TV and media player (e.g., DVD) is helpful for providing ready access to educational materials. These items should be secured in the room.

The offices of individual providers should be well insulated or at least have white-noise devices to prevent conversations from being overheard in the hallways or adjoining offices. If there is a desk in the office, it should not be a barrier between the patient and provider when talking. The room should have a window so that the supervisor or other staff can look in, a panic button, and easy access to the exit in case the patient becomes angry and/or violent. Places where the provider can secure valuables and confidential files should be provided (Bailes & Lowery, 2006).

Maintaining the Exterior and Interior of the Clinic With Limited Financial Resources

In reality, most treatment programs for patients with substance use disorders have quite limited financial resources to devote to clinic environment maintenance and upkeep. However, such a lack of funds should not prevent the staff from creating and maintaining a neat, tidy, clean, and inviting space. Small fundraisers can include bake sales or arts and crafts sales, with the arts and crafts made by the patients and staff. Volunteer days can be scheduled where the patients and staff come together to paint, weed, and pick up trash and debris. These activities can not only improve clinic maintenance but also foster respect for and ownership in the program.

Set Rules and Regulations

For the most part, having written rules provides a clear set of expectations for patients and helps staff members enforce them uniformly. These expectations of behavior should be provided in a written handbook that is given to the patient upon her admittance to treatment at the clinic. They should also be reviewed verbally with the patient, and the patient should sign and date them to acknowledge her agreement. Reviewing the rules communicates that they are important, that they are taken seriously, and that the clinic staff are professionals. The rules should also be posted on the back of the door of each group room and each clinic office. An example of some of the written rules that are provided as a part of a comprehensive treatment center is included in Appendix 3.1. The rules should be written in neutral or positive rather than punitive and negative language.

HOW TO GET AN ACCURATE ASSESSMENT OF YOUR CLINIC'S "ATMOSPHERE OF REINFORCEMENT"

One of the best ways to accurately assess the level of reinforcement of your clinic's atmosphere is to determine what it is like to be a patient in your organization or on your caseload. Conducting a walk-through with a group of clinic team members that include individuals from all levels of the organization, staff from other programs, and patient representatives can be enlightening to see both the program's positive aspects and the areas for improvement. Try to actively address any issues that create negative patient and staff experiences. The regular use of satisfaction surveys and focus groups asking about the access to aspects of treatment, the treatment itself, the staff who provide it, and the facility in which treatment is provided can be helpful for monitoring performance and improvement over time. Data should be collected from current patients as well as graduates and current and former staff to fully evaluate the clinic atmosphere. An example of items and a checklist that could be used in a comprehensive treatment program for pregnant patients with substance use disorders can be found in Appendix 3.2.

Finally, the Network for the Improvement of Addiction Treatment (NIATx) process improvement model (www.niatx.net) has a comprehensive approach designed to improve access to and engagement in treatment. Their model can serve as an excellent resource in the development and implementation of a comprehensive treatment program for pregnant patients with substance use disorders. The NIATx model is outlined in Table 3.1.

SUMMARY

Patient-centered care and effective treatment of women with substance use disorders while pregnant share the same basic foundation of forming a relationship. This relationship must be one that the patient feels that she would like to establish and maintain. Practical keys like keeping your word, active listening, positive attitudes, patience, and monitoring of the clinical environment will help ensure a positive atmosphere of reinforcement so that patients and the clinic providers and staff have respectful, supported, and affirming experiences while at the treatment setting.

Table 3-1. THE NIATx MODEL

Founded in 2003, the Network for the Improvement of Addiction Treatment (NIATx) is currently located at the University of Wisconsin–Madison's Center for Health Enhancement Systems (CHESS). The NIATx process model was developed to help substance use treatment programs enhance their policies and procedures so that such changes lead to improvements in patient access to and retention in treatment.

The NIATx model consists of *Four Aims*, *Five Principles*, *Promising Practices*, and the *Learning Collaborative*.

The Four Aims
1. Reduce waiting times for treatment admission.
2. Reduce no-shows for appointments.
3. Increase admissions to treatment.
4. Increase continuation in treatment.

The Five Principles
1. Understand and involve the customer.
2. Fix the key problems.
3. Pick a powerful change leader.
4. Get ideas from outside the organization or field.
5. Use rapidcycle testing to establish effective changes.

Promising Practices
Promising Practices provides a compilation of ideas that have fostered organizational change in a variety of treatment settings.

Learning Collaborative
The Learning Collaborative allows NIATx users to share ideas and services to improve their organizations. Services include coaching from members of other organizations and the NIATx website: www.niatx.net

---

(adapted from www.niatx.net)

REFERENCES

Ahire, D. (2007, October 5). Available online: http://www.buzzle.com/articles/good-customer-service-tips.html (accessed July 29, 2012).

Bailes, M., & Lowery, C. (2006), Practical issues of program organization and operation. In E. C. Strain & M. L. Stitzer (Eds.), *The treatment of opioid dependence* (pp. 178–212). Baltimore: Johns Hopkins University Press.

Najavits, L. M., & Weiss, R. D. (1994). Variations in therapist effectiveness in the treatment of patients with substance use disorders: An empirical review. *Addictions*, 89, 679–688.

Tahir, L. (2012). 10 customer service tips. Available online: http://sbinfocanada.about.com/od/customerservice/a/custservtipslt.htm (accessed October 22, 2012).

Ward, S. (2008). 8 rules for good customer service good customer service made simple. Available online: http://sbinfocanada.about.com/od/customerservice/a/custservrules.htm (accessed July 29, 2012).

APPENDIX 3-1. EXAMPLE OF WRITTEN RULES FOR A COMPREHENSIVE TREATMENT CENTER

The *mission of* the treatment program is to....[program would fill this in]
The *benefits* of the treatment clinic
Examples include:

- Having an individual counselor to assist me in my recovery
- Being able to access educational groups that cover key elements to help me build a drug-free life
- Having regular urine testing to confirm that I am free of drugs
- Having a process and procedure to appropriately address a urine test result that I think is incorrect
- Having a process and procedure to appropriately address an issue that I may have with another patient or a program staff person

With these benefits of treatment, I agree to and understand the following *responsibilities* that I have as a patient member of the treatment clinic. Examples include:

- Allowing myself and my personal items to be searched at any time while in treatment
- Free of carrying illicit or abused licit drugs or alcohol while on clinic property
- Free of carrying weapons or items that could be used as weapons while on clinic property
- I will not steal or harm anything that belongs to others
- I will not be verbally or physically violent against anyone
- I will give random samples of my *own* urine and blood for drug screens as requested by my treatment team
- I understand that if I break any of the above rules I *may* be discharged from the program

Explanation of the grievance process should be outlined to the patient in writing. Patient and provider both sign and date the form as acknowledging the benefits and responsibilities have been reviewed and are agreed to be followed.

APPENDIX 3-2. EXAMPLE ITEMS AND CHECKLIST FOR EVALUATION OF THE ATMOSPHERE AT A COMPREHENSIVE TREATMENT PROGRAM

Physical Structure of the Building

OUTSIDE
- Painting needed? specify area: _____
- Cigarette butts on ground?
- Landscaping tidy?
- Trash visible?
- Trash cans available and empty?
- Signage clear to tell visitors the name of the clinic and how to access it?
- Hours of operation posted?
- Any areas where people could hide?
- Lighting at night?
- Loitering rules posted?
- Security cameras in good working order?

INSIDE
- Painting needed? specify area: _____
- Safety mirrors needed? specify area: _____
- Educational materials available to patients?
- Bulletin board updated with recent information about health or social issues?
- Any areas that need safety improvements?
  specify area: _____

Focus Group and/or Secret Patient Questions

SHORTLY AFTER INTAKE
1. What did you like best about the intake process?
2. What could we do to make the intake process better?
3. Did you receive directions to get to the clinic for your intake?
4. Did you receive directions to locate the room of the clinic for your intake?
5. Was information given to you explaining each step of the intake process?
6. How often were you asked the same questions at intake?
   Not at all   /   2 or 3 times   /   4 or 5 times   /   6 or more times
7. How did the nature of information-gathering make you feel?

8. Did any questions on the part of [insert a process like intake or insert a division of treatment] lead you to feel stigmatized? If so, which ones:

    _____

9. How adequate was the information about the treatment and what to expect in the treatment?
   Not at all   /   a little bit   /   somewhat   /   pretty much   /   very much   /   not applicable

10. How much have you felt *cared about* by the clinic staff?
    Not at all   /   a little bit   /   somewhat   /   pretty much   /   very much   /   not applicable

11. Who has made you feel most welcome so far?

Other comments?

During Treatment

1. What do you like best about the treatment process?
2. What could we do to make the treatment process better?
3. What do you like best about the physical environment of the clinic?
4. What could we do to make the physical environment of the clinic better?
5. What treatment plans do you have after discharge?
6. Are there any treatment team members about whom you would like to say something positive? _____

Other comments?

At Treatment Discharge

1. What did you like best about the treatment process?
2. What could we have done to make the treatment process better?
3. What treatment plans do you have after discharge?
4. Are there any treatment team members that you would like to say something positive about? _____

Other comments?

A Step-by-Step Process for Identifying, Assessing, and Treatment Planning for Women with Substance Use Disorders During Pregnancy

Identifying Substance Use Disorders in the Pregnant Patient

OVERVIEW

Chapters 1 through 3 focused on general macro-level topics such as legal, ethical, theoretical, and contextual issues that provide a foundation for the second section of the book. Section II (Chapters 4 through 7) discusses the identification of, assessment of, and treatment planning for women with substance use disorders during pregnancy.

In this chapter we cover issues related to the identification and screening of pregnant women who may be at risk for substance use disorders and who may need treatment for these types of illnesses. The issues that will be presented include the benefits of screening, barriers to screening and methods to overcome them, types of screening (including self-report and biological measures), keys to selecting an appropriate screening instrument for the clinical setting in which pregnant women are seen, roles and responsibility of the provider in screening, and tips for facilitating referral for assessment, diagnosis, and treatment. A summary of the key points is presented at the end of the chapter.

INTRODUCTION

Women who use substances while they are pregnant may come into contact with multiple providers in the community, including first-aid workers, family medicine providers, nurses, primary care physicians, obstetrical care providers, and emergency department personnel, to name just a few examples. Early identification of substance use disorders in pregnant women can allow for intervention and treatment to minimize the potential harm to mother and child associated with untreated use of licit or illicit drugs. The American Congress of Obstetricians and Gynecologists (ACOG, 2004, 2006) recommends that all pregnant women be carefully and sensitively questioned about licit and illicit substance use. These substances should include prescription opioids and other medications that could be misused (ACOG, 2012). Further, every woman seeking obstetrical and/or gynecological services should be screened for alcohol use at least once every 12 months and within the first 13 weeks of pregnancy (ACOG, 2011).

Given the current state of the medical system in the United States, many factors hinder the ability and willingness of providers to screen pregnant women for substance use. Efforts are needed to change the health care system to make it more patient-, family-, and community-focused, as well as to promote rather than discourage providers from screening pregnant patients for substance use.

As an introduction to this chapter, it is important to define what we mean by the term *screening*. Screening is the process of identification of a patient who may be at risk for having a problem, in this case a health-related problem. Screening is only the first step in determining if a patient has a specific problem. Screening measures often cast a wider net and identify those individuals at risk who do not necessarily have a health-related problem. Screening for substance use risk typically places a patient in one of three categories: no risk, at risk for a substance use disorder, or clearly has the clinical indications of a substance use disorder. For those women without risk, no follow-up is necessary. Women at risk for a substance use disorder should be referred for assessment. Patients who clearly show signs of a substance use disorder should immediately be referred to treatment. At treatment entry, patients would receive an in-depth assessment of their substance use disorder and other areas in their lives that might be affected by their substance use.

Screening should be conducted only if the results will be acted upon, if indicated. Although multiple instruments are available for identifying individuals at risk for substance use, many of them have not been studied or validated in pregnant women. Also, there should be a good match between the provider setting and the screening instrument. Training in how to administer the instrument as well as how to respond to positive and negative results is needed so that screening can identify potential risks for substance use disorders without stigmatizing the patient.

BENEFITS OF SCREENING

Early detection of a substance use problem can lead to intervention and treatment, minimizing harm and improving outcomes for both mother and child.

As a part of the screening process, patients can receive education about the risks of alcohol, tobacco, and illicit drugs, as well as ways that they can improve their health and the well-being and health of the fetus.

BARRIERS TO SCREENING AND SUGGESTIONS FOR OVERCOMING THEM

One barrier to screening is the limited time that providers have to meet with each patient; time is limited because clinics need to see many patients due to the low reimbursement they receive for each individual patient. Other barriers to screening are lack of training or experience in screening, assessment, and intervention skills; the pessimistic attitude that identification will not lead to either treatment or behavior change; apprehension that there is no place or mechanism to refer patients if additional assessment and treatment are needed; fear that the patient will be offended and leave (see Svikis & Reid-Quiñones, 2003, for a review); fear of legal or ethical issues surrounding the identification of an at-risk patient; and uncertainty about how to address a positive screen. Each barrier and a potential method for overcoming it are discussed in the following section.

Lack of Provider Time for Screening

The time issue can be addressed on multiple fronts. The time it takes to administer the screening instrument can be reduced by using a computerized screening method that is completed in the waiting room, with the answer summary and scoring printed for the provider. Another option is to have the patient complete a self-administered screen in the waiting room before the visit; the staff member escorting the patient to the exam room can score the measure.

Lack of Provider Time for Addressing a Positive Screen Response

An obstetrical care provider once said, "Why would I want to screen for substance use in my patients? If it is there, then I have to take time away from activities that I get reimbursed for to do something about it. Honestly, other than a urine tox screen, I do not know how to screen her…then [I do not know] where to send a drug-addicted pregnant patient to get help." This example illustrates the fear and frustration providers feel when a screening result is positive. One way to ease the concern is to have both a checklist and a referral list of assessment places as part of the medical charting documents that will walk the provider through the steps needed to address this issue. Within 5 minutes, the provider could thank the patient for her honest disclosure and state that the next step is referral. The provider could explain that the patient will be referred for a more in-depth assessment and understanding of her substance use. Having a list of referral sources in the chart materials that can be given to the patient at the time of the visit and having a designated staff member to make the referral appointment and provide follow-up as needed will reduce both time and fear on the part of the provider and increase the number of women being screened for substance use.

Lack of Training in Screening

As illustrated in the quote from the provider above, training in screening for substance use during pregnancy is not always a part of medical school training. One way to address this issue is to let the provider and staff know that obtaining training may count as part of the continuing education credits needed for license renewal. Another option is the use of computerized screening tools; however, some staff training in how to interpret and address a positive screening result is still required.

Pessimistic Attitude That Identification Will Not Lead to Eventual Behavior Change

Another medical care provider once said: "What is the use of screening them for substance use anyway? It is not like knowing they are using and telling them to stop is going to do any good." This quote is an excellent example of the need to educate health care providers about substance use disorders and the effective treatments that are available. As discussed in Chapter 2, there are no "cures" for substance use disorders, but there are efficacious treatments. The earlier the problem is identified, the sooner treatment can begin. Being able to provide lists of assessment and treatment facilities and having the provider task clinical support staff as the referral point of contact may also increase the opportunity for the patient to receive care for this issue.

Apprehension That There Is Not a Place or Mechanism to Refer Positively Screened Patients for Additional Assessment and Treatment

One way to address these issues is to have designated staff address positive screening results and provide referrals. Another way is to have the computerized screen provide a printed list of referrals for assessment to patients meeting the criteria cutoff for a positive screening test result.

Fear of Legal or Ethical Issues

Another fear that providers have regarding screening for substance use in pregnant patients is that they may be required to call legal authorities or breach patient confidentiality and then have a patient leave treatment. Providers can be educated about the legal mandates and laws of confidentiality and mandated reporting regarding substance use in pregnant patients in their state. For each type of clinical practice there are ethical guidelines to help the provider determine the best course of action in this situation.

TYPES OF SCREENING INSTRUMENTS

Before discussing the different screening instruments, we should note that there is no one optimal screening tool for identifying which pregnant women are using substances (Wong et al., 2011). However, there are different types of screening tools that are helpful for identifying women using substances during pregnancy.

Screening Instruments Based on Self-Report

Maternal interviews using open-ended, nonjudgmental questions are likely to elicit disclosure of perinatal substance use (Hinderliter & Zelenak, 1993; Washington State Department of Health, Maternal and Child Health, 2012). While this is a common approach, there are structured and validated tools available. Most self-report screening instruments are in the form of questionnaires that are designed to be administered, in person, to the patient by the provider. What is becoming more popular is the use of computerized screening that could include audio-assisted computerized assessment (ACASI). Computerized screening for substance use disorders has been found to be well accepted by pregnant patients and yields valid information regarding substance use and other risk factors for negative pregnancy outcomes (Lapham et al., 1993). Potential advantages of computerized screening include (1) the reduced amount of provider time needed to administer the screen, (2) the increased anonymity patients feel when they do not have to answer potentially stigmatizing questions to a provider face to face —and thereby the more accurate answers they may provide, and (3) the ability to collect more detailed information than is easily obtained by paper forms (Satre et al., 2008).

Screening Instruments Not Based on Self-Report

Although laboratory tests and urine or other biological (e.g., saliva, urine) toxicology studies can be used in many cases to detect relatively recent substance use, a laboratory result by itself is an incomplete and ineffective method for determining a substance use disorder. Using hair to detect substance use offers a longer window of detection, but practical issues such as hair collection, the type of treatments the hair has received, the length of hair, and the cost of the test can be obstacles to its routine use. Blood- or breath-alcohol content and biological markers found in blood samples such as gamma-glutamyltransferase (GGT), aspartate aminotransferase (AST), erythrocyte mean corpuscular volume, and carbohydrate-deficient transferrin (CDT) have been used to determine heavy alcohol consumption (Das et al., 2008). Of these markers, CDT is the only test approved by the U.S. Food and Drug Administration for the identification of heavy alcohol use. When CDT and GGT are used together, the combination of results enhances the sensitivity of detection of heavy alcohol consumption, especially in clinical populations (Anton, 2001). However, women as a group produce more CDT under natural conditions and may produce less CDT in response to heavy drinking (Anton, 2001). Also, pregnant women produce more CDT over the course of the pregnancy, which may limit the diagnostic accuracy of this test during pregnancy (Stauber et al., 1996). Most biological makers, especially those measured in blood samples, may indicate heavy but not lighter alcohol use and will revert to normal levels following abstinence from alcohol for a few days up to a few weeks. Some patients with hazardous alcohol use will have normal test results, and some with less-risky drinking will have elevated results (Das et al., 2008). For cigarette smoking and illicit substance use, urine and in some cases, saliva tests, have been developed to detect recent use. Not all drug panels test for all drugs that can be abused. Further, within a testing class, not all drugs in that class will be detected with every test. For example, within the opioid class of drugs, there will need to be separate tests for methadone, OxyContin, and buprenorphine. Thus, care needs to be taken in determining which specific drugs are commonly abused and which drugs should be tested for in a specific clinical setting. For each substance and type of testing, there are different periods of detection and cutoff levels. The test results can be influenced by the type of substance used (some prescription medications will not be detected), the amount, frequency, rate of metabolism, route of administration, and recency of use. Also, some over-the-counter or prescribed medications may result in false-positive tests for illicit drugs. For example, common nasal decongestants can cause a positive reading for amphetamines; Vicks Formula 44M containing dextromethorphan, Primatene-M containing perylamine, the pain reliever Demerol, and the prescription antidepressant amitriptyline (Elavil) can produce urine screening results positive for opiates.

Other Indications of Risk for Substance Use During Pregnancy

Given the stigma of admitting to substance use and the fear of legal ramifications, women may not provide an accurate picture of their substance use. Thus, awareness of the other potential clinical indicators (Fig. 4.1) that are associated with substance use may help the provider determine the need for additional screening or assessment of substance use disorders during pregnancy.

FEATURES OF SUCCESSFUL SCREENING INSTRUMENTS AND SUCCESSFUL IMPLEMENTATION OF THESE INSTRUMENTS

The most effective screening instruments for substance use disorders are those that can be completed in less than 10 minutes; are performed with all patients; can be adapted to the provider's setting; have questions that assume that all patients use alcohol, smoke cigarettes, and use drugs by asking about quantity and frequency rather than the presence or absence of such use; and are repeated at each provider visit or at least at each trimester. Also, the screening questions should be embedded in other items asking about health behaviors (Institute of Medicine, 1990; Morse et al., 1997; Svikis et al., 2003). Health care providers should be aware of the other risk factors to inform their clinical impression in combination with the screener (Sarkar et al., 2009). Patients are usually not offended by questions about alcohol, cigarette, and substance use if they are asked in a neutral, caring, nonjudgmental, nonthreatening manner, and if the health implications and benefits of reduction and abstinence are stressed. All staff must understand the reasons for asking about substance use, even those who may not be involved in the actual interview. This open flow of information helps reduce bias from different staff members that may inadvertently be conveyed to patients. The provider needs to be ready to respond to questions from the patient or family or friends attending the appointment with the patient about why these questions are being asked. One way of normalizing the presentation of these questions is to embed them in other health behavior questions and preface the questions by stating that all patients are asked questions

Behavior Patterns
- Agitation
- Aggression
- Anxiety
- Cigarette smoking
- Depression
- Disorientation
- Euphoria
- Hallucinations
- Increased physical activity
- Intoxication (nodding, slurred speech, lack of coordination)
- Irritability
- Marijuana use may indicate other illicit drug use
- Nervousness
- Paranoia
- Prescription drug seeking behavior
- Rapid speech
- Repeated behaviors (e.g., constantly twisting hair, picking or scratching her skin)
- Suicidal ideations/attempt
- Sedation

Physical Signs

Eyes
- Dilated or constricted pupils
- Rapid eye movements

Nose
- Red/eroded nasal mucosa, nose bleeds

Mouth
- Gum or periodontal disease
- Skin conditions: abscesses, dry or itchy, acne type sores

Extremities and Skin
- Tremors
- Track marks or abscesses/injection sites

Vital Signs
- Clinically concerning increased or decreased pulse and blood pressure
- Increased body temperature
- Weight loss-low Body Mass Index (BMI)

Medical History
- Many events (numerous hospitalizations; wounds from weapons, infections)

Internal Organs and Chronic Medical Issues
- Liver problems (cirrhosis, hepatitis)
- Pancreatitis
- Diabetes
- Falls and bruises

Figure 4.1 Other Potential Indications of Risk for Substance Use during Pregnancy (Adapted from Washington State Department of Health, Maternal and Child Health, 2012)

such as these in order to obtain a complete picture of the patient's health and the health of her fetus (Washington State Department of Health, Maternal and Child Health, 2012).

Screening Instruments for Alcohol

There are more instruments for screening for alcohol use than for other drugs. Commonly used instruments include the CAGE (an acronym for the questions asking about *c*utting down alcohol; *a*nnoyed by being criticized for use of alcohol; feeling *g*uilty about behaviors when under the influence of alcohol; and having a drink after waking, *e*ye-opener) (e.g., Steinweg & Worth, 1993), the Michigan Alcoholism Screening Test (MAST; Selzer 1971), and the Alcohol Use Disorders Identification Test (AUDIT; Babor et al., 2001). While these are the most traditional screening instruments used in nonpregnant patients, the T-ACE (Sokol et al., 1989) and the TWEAK (Chang et al., 1999) are two questionnaires specifically developed and validated for screening for risky alcohol use in pregnant women. Both of these instruments have been found to be acceptable for use by pregnant women. The six-question CRAFFT instrument, which asks about issues such as riding in a car with someone under the influence, using substances to relax, using substances alone, and family or friends telling the woman to cut down, has been validated in pregnant adolescents (Chang et al., 2011).

Screening Instruments for Substance Use or Combined Alcohol and Substance Use

Instruments developed to screen for both alcohol and substance use in non-pregnant patients include the CAGE-AID (Brown & Rounds, 1995) the Drug Abuse Screening Test (DAST; Skinner, 1982; Skinner & Goldberg, 1986; Yudko et al., 2007), and the MAST/AD (Westermeyer et al., 2004). A few instruments have been developed for parenting and pregnant women. Of these instruments, there is a six-item combination of the DAST and MAST that was useful for detecting substance use in a pediatric clinic setting (Kemper et al., 1993). The 4Ps Plus asks about alcohol and substance use and was designed for pregnant women. It has a total of five questions in four areas: substance use problems in the patient's partner, in her parents, and at an earlier point in her, and use prior to pregnancy awareness. One endorsement of any question is considered a positive screen. The 4P's Plus has been reported to be reliable and valid (Chasnoff & Hung, 1999). The ALPHA tool, another option for providers, is a comprehensive instrument that includes CAGE-type questions to screen for maternal substance use within validated questions to identify associated psychosocial risk factors such as family violence or postpartum depression (Carroll et al., 2005; Reid et al., 1998).

SELECTION OF A SCREENING INSTRUMENT OR INSTRUMENTS

There are several aspects to consider when selecting a screening instrument for substance use in pregnant patients. The instrument needs to be one that the provider or staff feel comfortable administering, that fits into the routine aspects of clinical care, and that screens for a wide variety of substances, including tobacco, alcohol, illicit drugs, and misuse of prescription medications. Screening instruments are only one part of the complete information needed to obtain a sensitive and accurate clinical picture of the patient's risk for substance use (e.g., Svikis et al., 2003).

ROLES AND RESPONSIBILITIES IN SCREENING

It is important for providers to know how to respond appropriately to a negative screen and a positive screen.

Negative Screens

If the screen is negative, providers should remember that all brief screening instruments rely on the respondent's honesty. Thus, providers may wish to discuss substance use with any patient whom they believe failed to respond honestly to the screening questions. For example, it may be important to ask questions such as: "I note you indicate you don't drink alcohol. Many women who become pregnant drank before they became pregnant. Did you? How difficult was it to quit drinking alcohol after you learned you were pregnant?" to attempt to ascertain the woman's truthfulness in responding. If the provider receives incomplete and/or conflicting answers, and thus has concerns on the basis of this interview, it may be appropriate to refer the patient for further assessment.

If the provider is confident that the patient has been honest and accurate in her responses, the following actions might be taken: (1) Praise the patient for her health-conscious approach to her pregnancy; (2) Review the benefits of continued abstinence from all substances during pregnancy; (3) Remind her to avoid even secondhand smoke.

Positive Screens

If the screen is positive for substance use, the following actions should be taken: (1) Thank the woman for her honest disclosure; (2) Remind her that you know as the mother she wants her baby to be as healthy as possible and that she can improve the health of her baby by discontinuing use of alcohol and drugs; (3) Suggest a referral for a more in-depth assessment by a specialist; and (4) If the in-depth assessment shows her behavior is risky, you, as the provider, will help her to stop using drugs and/or alcohol; she is not alone in this effort—and the first step in this process is referral for assessment of the extent of the illness. Ideally, the referral and appointment for the assessment should be made while the patient is in the office.

TIPS FOR FACILITATING REFERRAL FOR ASSESSMENT, DIAGNOSIS, AND TREATMENT

If you are having trouble finding clinics or service delivery providers where you can refer patients for assessment and treatment, try your state's Division of Substance Abuse Services; ask for a list of referral agencies. Ideally, pregnant women should be assessed and treated for substance use disorders in a specialty program tailored to women and pregnancy, but not all states or communities have these types of programs. There are private hospitals, psychiatrists, psychologists, and counselors who treat substance use disorders. Twelve Step programs such as Alcoholics (or Cocaine or Narcotics) Anonymous can also provide useful support to women seeking help for these problems. All of these programs are usually listed in the phone book and on the Internet.

Once an appointment for assessment or treatment is set, the provider or the provider's staff should follow up with the patient to see if she kept the appointment and then either praise her for keeping this appointment or actively work with her to reschedule the appointment. Praise any reduction in use that she reports to you—do not reserve praise for abstinence-only behavior. If the assessment determines she needs treatment, maintain communication with the treatment provider to monitor progress.

Regardless of how far along a patient is in her pregnancy, emphasize that the benefits of identification and treatment will begin as soon as she reduces or stops use, and that the earlier she is able to do so the better. It is never too late to start to make positive changes in her health behavior, however.

SUMMARY

All pregnant women should be carefully, sensitively, and confidentially questioned about licit and illicit substance use at multiple times during their pregnancy—asking once is not enough. Early identification of substance use disorders in pregnant women can allow for intervention and treatment to minimize the potential harms to mother, fetus, and child that are associated with untreated use of licit or illicit drugs. Screening for substance use is important and can be done efficiently and without taking away valuable clinical time. Screening for substance use should include not only a questionnaire but also a clinical evaluation and determination of the need for further assessment. Several instruments that screen for both alcohol and drugs and instruments have been designed for pregnant women. In the absence of a head-to-head comparison of these combination measures, each provider should select the instrument that he or she is most comfortable using. Knowing how to respond effectively to negative screens and positive screens is critical so that patients can continue their healthy behaviors or consider making behavioral changes.

REFERENCES

American College of Obstetricians and Gynecologists. (2004). Committee Opinion Number 294: At-risk drinking and illicit drug use. Ethical Issues In Obstetric and Gynecologic Practice.

American College of Obstetricians and Gynecologists. (2006). Committee Opinion No. 343: Psychosocial Risk Factors: Perinatal Screening and Intervention.

American College of Obstetricians and Gynecologists. (2011). Committee Opinion 496: At-risk drinking and alcohol dependence: Obstetric and gynecologic implications. *Obstetrics & Gynecology, 118*(2 Pt 1), 383–388.

American Congress of Obstetricians and Gynecologists. (2012). Committee Opinion 524: Opioid abuse, dependence and addiction in pregnancy. Available online: http://www.acog.org/~/media/Committee%20Opinions/Committee%20on%20Health%20Care%20for%20Underserved%20Women/co524.pdf?dmc=1&ts=20120504T063446 4326 (accessed July 28, 2012).

Anton, R. F. (2001). Carbohydrate-deficient transferrin for detection and monitoring of sustained heavy drinking. What have we learned? Where do we go from here? *Alcohol, 25*(3), 185–188.

Babor, T. F., de la Fuente J. R., Saunders, J., & Grant, M . (2001). *AUDIT: The Alcohol Use Disorders Identification Test.* Guidelines for Use in Primary Health Care (2nd ed., pp. 1–40). Geneva, Switzerland.

Brown, R. L. & Rounds, L. A. (1995). Conjoint screening questionnaires for alcohol and other drug abuse: criterion validity in a primary care practice. *Wisconsin Medical Journal, 94*(3), 135–140.

Carroll, J. C., Reid, A. J., Biringer, A., Midmer, D., Glazier, R. H., Wilson, L., et al. (2005). Effectiveness of the Antenatal Psychosocial Health Assessment (ALPHA) form in detecting psychosocial concerns: A randomized controlled trial. *Canadian Medical Association Journal, 173,* 253–259.

Chang, G., Wilkins-Haug, L., Berman, S., & Goetz, M. A . (1999). The TWEAK: application in a prenatal setting. *Journal of Studies on Alcohol, 60,* 306–310.

Chang, G ., Orav, E. J., Jones, J. A., et al. (2011). Self-reported alcohol and drug use in pregnant young women: a pilot study of associated factors and identification. *Journal of Addiction Medicine, 5,* 221–226.

Chasnoff, I. J., & Hung, W. C . (1999). *The 4P's Plus.* Chicago: NTI Publishing.

Chasnoff, I. J., Wells, A. M., McGourty, R. F., & Bailey, L. K. (2007). Validation of the 4P's Plus screen for substance use in pregnancy validation of the 4P's Plus. *Journal of Perinatology, 27*(12), 744–748.

Das, S. K., Dhanya, L., & Vasudevan, D. M . (2008). Biomarkers of alcoholism: an updated review. *Scandinavian Journal of Clinical and Laboratory Investigation, 68,* 81–92.

Hinderliter, S. A., & Zelenak, J. P. (1993). A simple method to identify alcohol and other drug use in pregnant adults in a prenatal care setting. *Journal of Perinatology, 13,* 93–102.

Institute of Medicine (1990). Who provides treatment? In Committee of the Institute of Medicine, Division of Mental Health and Behavioral Medicine (Ed.), *Broadening the base of treatment for alcoholism* (pp. 98–141). Washington D.C.: National Academy Press.

Kemper, K. J., Greteman, A., Bennett, E., & Babonis, T. R . (1993). Screening mothers of young children for substance abuse. *Journal of Development & Behavioral Pediatricts, 14*(5), 308–312.

Lapham, S. C., Henley, E., & Kleyboecker, K . (1993). Prenatal behavioral risk screening by computer among Native Americans. *Family Medicine Journal, 25*(3),197–202.

Morse, B., Gehshan, S., & Hutchins, E . (1997). *Screening for substance abuse during pregnancy: Improving care, improving health.* Arlington, VA: National Center for Education in Maternal and Child Health.

Reid, A. J., Biringer, A., Carroll, J. D., Midmer, D., Wilson, L. M., Chalmers, B., et al. (1998). Using the ALPHA form in practice to assess antenatal psychosocial health: Antenatal psychosocial health assessment. *Canadian Medical Association Journal, 159,* 677–684.

Sarkar, M., Burnett, M., Carrière, S., Cox, L. V., Dell, C. A., Gammon, H., Geller, B., Koren, G., Lee, L., Midmer, D., Mousmanis, P., Schuurmans, N., Senikas, V., Soucy, D., & Wood, R . (2009). Screening and recording of alcohol use among women of child-bearing age and pregnant women. *Canadian Journal of Clinical Pharmacology, 16*(1), 242–263.

Satre, D., Wolfe, W., Eisendrath, S., & Weisner, C . (2008). Computerized screening for alcohol and drug use among adults seeking outpatient psychiatric services. *Psychiatric Services*, *59*, 441–444.

Selzer, M. L . (1971). The Michigan Alcoholism Screening Test: the quest for a new diagnostic instrument. *American Journal of Psychiatry*, *127*(12), 1653–1658.

Skinner, H. A . (1982). The Drug Abuse Screening Test. *Addictive Behaviors*, *7*, 363–371.

Skinner, H. A., & Goldberg, A. E. (1986). Evidence for a drug dependence syndrome among narcotic users. *British Journal of Addiction*, *81*, 471–484.

Sokol, R. J., Martier, S. S., & Ager, J. W . (1989). The T-ACE questions: Practical prenatal detection of risk drinking. *American Journal of Obstetrics and Gynecology*, *160*(4), 863–870.

Stauber, R. E., Jauk, B., Fickert, P., & Häusler, M . (1996). Increased carbohydrate-deficient transferring during pregnancy: relation to sex hormones. *Alcohol*, *31*(4), 389–392.

Steinweg, D. L., & Worth, H . (1993). Alcoholism: The keys to the CAGE. *American Journal of Medicine*, *94*, 520–523.

Svikis, D. S., & Reid-Quiñones, K . (2003).Screening and prevention of alcohol and drug use disorders in women. *Obstetrics and Gynecology Clinics of North America*, *30*(3), 447–468.

Washington State Department of Health, Maternal and Child Health (2012). *Substance abuse during pregnancy: guidelines for screening (Rev. ed.).* http://here.doh.wa.gov/materials/guidelines-substance-abuse-pregnancy/15_PregSubs_E12L.pdf (accessed October 16, 2012).

Westermeyer, J., Yargic, I., & Thuras, P . (2004). Michigan Assessment-Screening Test for Alcohol and Drugs (MAST/AD): evaluation in a clinical sample. *American Journal on Addictions*, *13*(2), 151–162.

Wong, S., Ordean, A., Kahan, M., and the Society of Obstetricians and Gynecologists of Canada. (2011). SOGC clinical practice guidelines: Substance use in pregnancy #256, April 2011. *International Journal of Gynaecology & Obstetrics*, *114*(2), 190–202.

Yudko, E., Lozhkina, O., & Fouts, A . (2007). A comprehensive review of the psychometric properties of the Drug Abuse Screening Test. *Journal of Substance Abuse Treatment*, *32*(2), 189–198.

Comprehensive Assessment of the Pregnant Patient with Substance Use Disorders

OVERVIEW

This chapter discusses the comprehensive array of problems that a woman with a substance use disorder brings to treatment and how this complex constellation of characteristics requires an all-inclusive assessment. We describe the need for assessments to be woman-centered to identify women's special needs and provide examples of specific types of questions. We discuss internal barriers such as stigma and partner dynamics and external barriers such as child care and transportation that often prevent women with substance use disorders from entering and engaging in treatment. We then emphasize how comprehensive assessment and understanding can reduce or eliminate such barriers. The chapter concludes with a summary that emphasizes the key points made in the chapter.

INTRODUCTION

The intake assessment must be comprehensive and relevant to the array of issues that women with substance use disorders bring to treatment. The literature has clearly established that this population has special needs and characteristics that must be acknowledged and addressed to successfully engage these women in treatment (Comfort & Kaltenbach, 1999). A comprehensive assessment is essential so that treatment can be tailored to build upon the woman's individual strengths and address her needs and those of her child.

ASSESSMENTS

Unfortunately, existing substance use assessment instruments have been developed and/or validated primarily on male patients. Even the most widely used instrument, the Addiction Severity Index (ASI), was initially tested with a population of male military veterans (McLellan et al., 1980). However, one of the primary reasons the ASI is so widely used is because of its multidimensional approach to evaluating substance use: not only does it assess the patient's drug and alcohol status, but it also examines medical, psychiatric, legal, employment/support, and family/social relationship areas. Poor functioning in any of these areas affects the severity of substance use. The fifth edition (McLellan et al., 1992) sought to address some of the initial limitations of the ASI in terms of its appropriateness for use with women by including questions on physical and sexual abuse and long-term personal relationships. This version has also been standardized with pregnant women. However, for a number of researchers/providers working specifically with pregnant women, the fifth edition is still deficient because it does not assess pregnancy status and history, housing and caregiving responsibilities for children, status of intimate relationships, and history of violence and victimization. Fortunately, the developers of the ASI have always stressed that their semistructured interview can be adapted to meet the informational needs of programs and have encouraged the development of supplemental questions that meet the needs of specific populations (McLellan, 1992, McLellan et al., 2006).

Programs can certainly develop their own biopsychosocial assessment, as long as it meets the needs of the clinical and administrative service delivery system in terms of requirements of state licensing entities, credentialing bodies in the case of opioid treatment programs, and behavioral health payers. We have chosen to use the ASI because of its widespread use in both clinical and research settings and the ability to add supplemental questions without violating the instrument's integrity.

Several research projects focused on treatment for women with substance use disorders have integrated new items into the ASI. The Families of Recovering Mothers project (FORM) added items to the ASI and used a separate housing and family interview (Comfort et al., 1991), and the Family Life ASI (Brown, 1990) added items to address pregnancy information. Comfort and Kaltenbach (1996) used a more extensive approach: they developed a comprehensive psychosocial assessment, the Psychosocial History (PSH), that includes areas relevant to barriers to treatment, women's needs and strengths, and substance use treatment outcomes. The ASI items adapted from the FORM ASI, and the Family Life ASI, were embedded within the PSH.

The PSH included numerous questions about family history and relationships, relationships with partner, responsibilities for children, current health problems, pregnancy history, substance use during pregnancy, perinatal medical status, previous treatment experiences, employment history, history of violence and victimization, housing arrangements, family legal issues, and current housing arrangements. The questions expanded the seven domains of the ASI and added sections that addressed pregnancy history, partner history, family history, child care, and housing arrangements. The psychometric properties of the PSH relative to the ASI have been evaluated (Comfort at al., 1999) and found to yield reliable and valid data similar to the ASI and to provide a more comprehensive assessment than the ASI in the areas of pregnancy, family issues, and victimization. Although the PSH provides extensive information, it is labor-intensive, requiring several hours for administration, and may have to be conducted over several assessment sessions. Accordingly, it may be less useful in a clinical setting than a more abbreviated expansion of the ASI.

A multisite clinical trial investigating the use of methadone and buprenorphine in the management of opioid dependence during pregnancy (Jones et al., 2010, 2012) added a few salient items to the ASI to capture issues critical for pregnant women. Examples include additional demographic information such as how many times the respondent has been pregnant, how many times a pregnancy has resulted in childbirth, with how many different persons the respondent has had children, and how old the respondent was when her first child was born. Medical history includes supplemental questions about how long ago the respondent's last obstetrical/gynecological exam was and whether she has been tested for HIV. The Family/Social domain expands questions on children to include children's living arrangements, caretaking of children on a regular basis other than the mother, and access to emergency or backup child care. Questions on emotional support are also included, such as how much the respondent feels cared about by the significant people in her life and the degree to which she feels she needs additional support. These examples give an idea of the scope of items that need to be included in a comprehensive assessment so that treatment can be individualized.

Depending on the extensiveness of the biopsychosocial assessment, programs may also want to supplement their intake assessment with specialized assessments. Specifically, the two areas that require evaluation are the presence of depression and a history of trauma. Many women with substance use disorder suffer from depression, but this is especially salient for pregnant women (Martin et al., 2009). Programs providing treatment to pregnant women for substance use disorders should assess for depression at a minimum on intake and between 4 and 6 weeks postpartum. The Beck Depression Inventory (BDI; Beck et al., 1996) is widely used to assess depression in nonpregnant and antepartum patients. Two instruments commonly used to identify women at risk for post-partum depression are the Edinburgh Postnatal Depression Scale (EPDS; Cox et al., 1987) and the Postpartum Depression Screening Scale (PDSS9; Beck & Gable, 2000). These screening tools may be administered by nonpsychiatric staff. Postpartum depression may be a significant factor in relapse if not ade-quately treated. If treatment programs do not include psychiatric services, they must provide a network of psychiatrists for consultation and referral.

The prevalence of trauma, including physical and sexual abuse as children, in the lives of women with substance use disorders is overwhelming (see Chapter 12 for a more detailed discussion). Traditionally, substance use treatment pro-grams have focused on a patient's need to be secure in his or her recovery before addressing issues related to trauma. However, as described in Chapter 12, it is now recognized that responding to the effects of trauma is essential to achieving recovery and that services must be provided within a trauma-informed envi-ronment (Substance Abuse Mental Health Administration, U.S. Department of Health and Human Services, 2012). To develop treatment plans for recovery, a history of trauma should be assessed as early in intake as clinically appropri-ate. For example, such an assessment would not be part of the initial intake but would be conducted by the provider after establishing a therapeutic rapport. It is important that clinical support be available should an assessment trigger an adverse event such as a flashback. Several trauma assessment tools, such as the Trauma Symptom Inventory (Briere et al., 1995), can be used to identify the degree of trauma a woman has experienced.

BARRIERS TO TREATMENT ACCESS AND ENGAGEMENT

Just as treatment for substance use disorders needs to employ a woman-centered program to address the woman's treatment needs, so too is a women-centered perspective necessary to reduce barriers for women entering and engaging in treatment. For pregnant women, the stigma of being addicted, the fear of losing custody of her child, and the threat of incarceration and/or being mandated to enter treatment often pose insurmountable barriers to her seeking treatment. Creating a treatment environment that is welcoming, nonjudgmental, and supportive is essential to overcoming such barriers. (A detailed discussion of such a positive treatment environment is included in Chapter 3.) While pro-grams and staff must always be clear that their responsibilities as health care providers mandate reporting to local or state authorities, they should provide the support, clinical services, and referrals necessary to eliminate or reduce the chances that the mother will need to be reported to child protective serv-ices (see Chapter 1).

Women who have partners with substance use disorders often face major barriers both in accessing and engaging in treatment. Their partners may not be supportive of their treatment seeking and may even threaten violence or abandonment if they enter treatment. If the woman persists and does enter treatment, this dynamic often continues, with the partner attempting to sabotage her progress in treatment. The program and the staff must be sensitive and responsive to the multiple issues of her safety, the demands and stress of her relationship, and the impact on her ability to successfully engage in treatment.

Lack of child care and transportation are often cited as the most significant external barriers that prevent women from accessing services (Brady & Ashley, 2005). Transportation can be provided by vans or by giving women tokens for public transportation. Women receiving public assistance may be eligible for monthly transportation passes. Eligibility verification, enrollment, and distribution of monthly passes can be facilitated by a case manager or other program support staff.

While there may be a critical need for child care services, providing these services is not always a simple solution. Women may be reluctant to accept child care services for numerous reasons, such as fear of being reported to child protective services, having little experience leaving their children in a formal child care setting, and not knowing and/or not trusting child care workers (Comfort et al., 2000). Resistance may be based on experiential or clinical issues—again underlining the complexity of treatment issues in these women's lives. Strategies to overcome resistance may include having child care staff participate in the program orientation, both to familiarize women with the child care services and to reinforce their position as members of the treatment team; inviting mothers to spend time in the child care center before bringing their children; partnering new patients with patient mentors who can answer questions and alleviate anxieties; and integrating parenting concerns into the clinical treatment plan. The child care services must be grounded in a gentle, caring, supportive environment, but one in which it is always clear that treatment providers are required to report abuse and neglect to child protective services.

Offering on-site child care services while mothers attend groups, individual therapy sessions, and medical appointments; providing classes to improve parenting skills; offering mother/child recreational activities such as trips to zoos, farms, etc.; and offering counseling support for the difficulties and stress associated with parenting can all help reduce barriers associated with child care.

In developing comprehensive services to address multiple needs, it is important to ask the women which services they find most helpful. It is not unusual for them to report that the most practical concrete services, such as transportation assistance and help obtaining food, housing, clothing, child care, etc., are the most useful (Nelson-Zlupko et al., 1996). Health care professionals must recognize that meeting the needs of everyday living goes hand in hand with successfully engaging pregnant and parenting women in treatment.

SUMMARY

Women with substance use disorders have a complex array of problems that require comprehensive, woman-centered assessments. Such assessments are necessary so that treatment can be individualized. Part of this comprehensive approach is providing practical services that reduce barriers to engagement and retention in treatment for pregnant women and women with young children.

REFERENCES

Beck, A. T., Steer, R. A., & Brown, G. K. (1996). *Beck Depression Inventory* (2nd ed.). San Antonio, TX: Psychological Corporation.

Beck, C. T., & Gable, R. K. (2000). Postpartum Depression Screening Scale: Development and psychometric testing. *Nursing Research, 49,* 272–282.

Brady, T. M., & Ashley, O. S. (Eds.) (2005). *Women in substance abuse treatment: Results from the Alcohol and Drug Services Study* (ADSS) (DHHS Publication No. SMA 04–3968, Analytic Series A-26). Rockville, MD, Substance Abuse and Mental Health Services Administration, Office of Applied Studies.

Briere, J., Elliott, D. M., Harris, K., & Cotman, A. (1995). Trauma Symptom Inventory: Psychometrics and association with childhood and adult trauma in clinical samples. *Journal of Interpersonal Violence, 10*(4), 387–401.

Brown, E. (1990). Maternal measures. Discussion conducted at the National Institute on Drug Abuse Perinatal-20 Treatment Research Demonstration Program Meeting, Bethesda, MD, November 9.

Comfort, M., & Kaltenbach, K. (1999). Biopsychosocial characteristics and treatment outcomes of pregnant cocaine-dependent women in residential and outpatient substance abuse treatment. *Journal of Psychoactive Drugs, 31*(3), 279–289.

Comfort, M., Richlin, L., Shipley, T. E., White, K., & Shandler, I. (1991). Final report of the F.O.R.M. Project. In *Treatment for drug-exposed women and their children: Advances in research methodology.* NIDA Research Monograph Series 166, pp. 123–142. Washington DC: U.S. Government Printing Office.

Comfort, M., Zanis, D.A., Whitely, M.J., Kelly-Tyler, A., & Kaltenbach, K. (1999). Assessing the needs of substance abusing women: psychometric data on the Psychosocial History. *Journal of Substance Abuse Treatment, 17*(1–2), 79–83.

Comfort, M. L., & Kaltenbach, K. (1996). The Psychosocial History: an interview for pregnant and parenting women in substance abuse treatment and research. In *Treatment for drug-exposed women and their children: Advances in research methodology.* NIDA Research Monograph Series 166, pp. 123–142. Washington DC: U.S. Government Printing Office.

Comfort, M. L., Loverro, J., & Kaltenbach, K. (2000). A search for strategies to engage women in substance abuse treatment. *Social Work in Health Care, 31*(4), 59–70.

Cox, J., Holden, J., & Sagovsky, R. (1987). Detection of postnatal depression: Development of the 10-item Edinburgh Postnatal Depression Scale. *British Journal of Psychiatry, 150,* 782–786.

Jones, H. E., Fischer, G., Heil, S. H., Kaltenbach, K., Martin, P. R., Coyle, M. G., Selby, P., Stine, O'Grady, K. E., & Arria, A. M. (2012). Maternal Opioid Treatment: Human Experimental Research (MOTHER): Approach, issues, and lessons learned. *Addiction, 107*(Suppl. 1), 28–35.

Jones, H. E., Kaltenbach, K., Heil, S. H., Stine, S. M., Coyle, M. G., Arria, A. M., O'Grady, K. E., Selby, P., Martin, P. R., & Fischer, G. (2010). Neonatal abstinence syndrome after methadone or buprenorphine exposure. *New England Journal of Medicine, 363*(24), 2320–2331.

Martin, P., Arria, A. M., Fischer, G., Kaltenbach, K., Heil, S., Stine, S., Coyle, M. G., Selby, P., & Jones, H. E. (2009). Psychopharmacologic management of opioid-dependent women during pregnancy. *American Journal on Addictions, 18*(2), 148–156.

McLellan, A. T. (1992, March). *Planning Committee Document for the ASI Technology Transfer Package.* Planning session for the National Institute on Drug Abuse ASI Training Package, Washington DC.

McLellan, A. T., Cacciola, J. C., Alterman, A. I., Rikoon, S. H., & Carise, D. (2006). The Addiction Severity Index at 25: origins, contributions and transitions. *American Journal of Addictions, 15*(2), 113–124.

McLellan, A. T., Kushner, H., Metzger, D., Peters, R., Smith, I., Grissom, G., Pettinati, H., & Argeriou, M. (1992). The fifth edition of the Addiction Severity Index. *Journal of Substance Abuse Treatment, 9,* 199–213.

McLellan, A. T., Luborsky, L., O'Brian, C. P., & Woody, G. E. (1980). An improved evaluation instrument for substance abuse patients: The Addiction Severity Index. *Journal of Nervous Mental Disease, 168,* 26–33.

Nelson-Zlupko, L., Dore, M. M., Kauffman, E., & Kaltenbach, K. (1996). Women in recovery. Their perceptions of treatment effectiveness. *Journal of Substance Abuse Treatment, 13*(1), 51–59.

Substance Abuse Mental Health Administration, National Center for Trauma Informed Care. Available online: www.samhsa.gov/nctic (accessed July 3, 2012).

6

Individualized Care Plan: Development, Initiation, Monitoring, and Completion

OVERVIEW

This chapter builds upon the information provided in Chapters 4 and 5. Chapter 4 discussed the instruments used to determine who is at risk for substance use during pregnancy and how to respond appropriately to the results. Chapter 5 reviewed ways to assess the many aspects of women's lives that are touched by substance use disorders. In this chapter we continue the theme of comprehensive assistance for treating substance use disorders during pregnancy by providing a step-by-step guide to developing a care plan. This guide includes measures to help providers monitor progress in all aspects of comprehensive care and also to prepare patients for discharge and treatment completion. A case vignette will be used to illustrate each aspect of this care plan. Topics for discussion include development, initiation, monitoring, and completion of the treatment plan. As with all chapters, the points of emphasis in the chapter are summarized.

FICTITIOUS CASE VIGNETTE

Felicia Jackson's life story is one of survival. On her 14th birthday, her present from her stepfather was an introduction to heroin. After a few exposures to heroin, he began sexually molesting her. At age 15, she ran away from home and lived on the street or with friends. To make money for food and shelter, she began prostituting herself and working in strip joints. She is now 30 and reports taking three alprazolam (Xanax) pills a day (benzodiazepines) and heroin (three injections, totaling $30/day) and smoking a pack of cigarettes a day.

She has three children, all in foster care. For this pregnancy, Felicia entered substance use treatment when she was 20 weeks pregnant, motivated by seeing her belly growing and the inability to deny any longer that she was pregnant. Felicia perceives this child as someone to finally "love me for me," and she wants to "do right by this baby this time." The pregnancy and expected child gives Felicia a reason to be "clean this time." The only time her substance use has been interrupted is by three prior incarcerations, two for commercial sex work and one for drug possession. She has an outstanding warrant for her arrest due to stabbing a "john." Felicia is currently anemic; she tests positive for hepatitis and negative for HIV. She has been afraid to seek obstetrical care for fear the staff will report her to the authorities and possibly take away her child at delivery. Felicia has three ongoing relationships with men with whom she exchanges sex for food, shelter, and other material goods. She arrives at the treatment clinic having taken a "small hit" of heroin to hold her over before she gets her methadone, which she has been told by other patients she will receive if she is using heroin. Felicia has evidence of track marks on her arms. Her urine sample was positive for both opioids and benzodiazepines. She screens positive for depression and anxiety disorders and has neither a stable living situation—she lives off and on with her three different partners—nor an adequate supply of food or physical security.

The fictional case of Felicia illustrates many of the challenges of developing and implementing a treatment plan for a pregnant woman with a substance use disorder and multiple life challenges. In her comprehensive assessment she provided the information above that will be key to determining her individualized treatment plan. Figure 6.1 (adapted from Jones et al., 2009) shows the key decisions that the treatment team will need to make in collaboration with Felicia.

DEVELOPING THE TREATMENT PLAN

The treatment plan is shown in Figure 6.2. Each part will be discussed below. This plan would be completed with the patient after the initial intake information is provided. As illustrated in the case vignette, Felicia has multiple issues that need to be concurrently addressed:

1. Survival needs: safe housing, free from others using drugs, and adequate food; could also include physical safety from a violent or abusing partner or family member

2. Psychiatric treatment: would always include treatment for substance use disorders and in appropriate cases, such as Felicia's, would include the treatment of comorbid psychiatric illnesses like depression and posttraumatic stress disorder

Treatment team
Counselor   Psychiatrist   Social Worker   Obstetrician   Lactation Consultant Pediatrician   Child Protective Service Worker

Treatment Plan Elements Based on Initial Assessment

☐**1 Survival**
  ☐Housing
  ☐Food

☐**2a Psychiatric Treatment for addiction**
  ☐Opioid agonist for heroin dependence
  ☐Medically-assisted withdrawal from benzos
  ☐Start nicotine cessation program

☐**2b Psychiatric Treatment of Co-Morbid Conditions**
  ☐Depression (medication and behavioral therapy)
  ☐Refer to PTSD and substance use disorder
    therapy
  ☐Select agonist medication for heroin dependence
  ☐Start individual and group counseling to address
    drug use

☐**3 Medical Treatment**
  ☐Hepatitis C medication
  ☐Iron for anemia
  ☐Regular prenatal laboratory testing

☐**4 Nutrition**
  ☐Initiate a food diary
  ☐Prenatal vitamin prescription and track
    adherence to ingestion
  ☐Nutrition education group

☐**5 Obstetrical Treatment**
  ☐Referral to OB
  ☐Track OB appointment
    attendance
  ☐Refer to OB education group
  *The **ideal** is referral to an OB
  with expertise in addiction
  medicine. However, the OB
  does not have to be an expert in
  addiction medicine.*

☐**6 Legal Assistance**
  ☐Help with outstanding
    warrannt

☐**7 Vocational Assistance**
  ☐Determine education or job
    goals

☐**8 Social Functioning**
  ☐Obtain NA sponsor
  ☐Track NA attendance
  ☐Couples therapy
  ☐HIV risk reduction skills
  ☐Stable drug-free housing

☐**9 Recreation**
  ☐Identify and practice drug-
    free fun activities

Key Decisions during Treatment

☐Opioid medication induction regimen
☐Medication-assisted withdrawal from benzos
☐Selection of an anti-depression medication
☐Selection of treatment regimen for PTSD
☐Selection of vocational/educational goal

☐Decision about remaining in current rela-
  tionships
☐How to build a drug-free peer network
☐Selection of NA sponsor
☐Decision to breastfeed
☐Decision regarding postpartum medication

Decisions to Prepare for Discharge

☐Opioid medication program transfer
☐Physician to transfer depression and anxiety management
☐Plan for continuing job maintenance behaviors
☐Plan to continue in parenting skills training

Figure 6.1 Treatment Team, Treatment Plan Elements, and Key Decisions

PROBLEM AREA (PRIORITY RANKING)	GOAL	INTERVENTION	OBJECTIVE MEASURE
1. Survival Needs			
1. Lack of safe housing	1. Recovery House	1. Live in Recovery House	1. Verify with house manager
2. Inadequate food	2. Food assistance	2. Go to Social Services	2. Self-report/bring in Social Services card
2a. Psychiatric Treatment: Substance Use Disorders			
1. Heroin use	1. Abstinence	1. Comprehensive treatment	1. Urine sample negative for heroin
1a. Benzodiazepine use	1a. Abstinence	1a. Medication assisted withdrawal	1a. Ingestion of less medication
			1a. Low benzo diazepine withdrawal scores
2. Nicotine	2. Abstinence	2. Nicotine replacement medication	2. Carbon monoxide less than 8 ppm
2b. Psychiatric Treatment: Comorbid Issues			
1. Depression (medication and behavioral therapy)	1. Controlled depression	1. SSRI (depression medication)	1. Low Beck Depression Inventory Scores
		1. Individual cognitive behavioral therapy	
2. PTSD	2. Controlled PTSD	2. PTSD and substance use group	2. Low scores on SCL-90
3. Medical			
1. Hepatitis C	1. Manage effects	1. Medication	1. Self-report and verify
		1. Liver function testing	1. Prescription given and filled
2. Anemia	2. Adequate iron	2.Daily iron ingestion	2. Self-report and verify prescription given and filled
		2. Prenatal blood testing	

Figure 6.2 Initial Treatment Plan

4. Nutrition			
1. Lack of nutrition	1. Balanced diet	1. Initiate a food diary	1. Track adherence to diary and ingestion of prenatal vitamin
		1. Prenatal vitamin prescription	
		1. Nutrition education group	
5. Obstetrical Treatment			
1. No prenatal care	1. Regular prenatal care	1. Referral to OB with addiction expertise	1. Track OB appointment attendance
		1. Refer to OB education group	1. Track OB education group attendance
6. Legal Assistance			
1. Warrant for arrest	1. No legal issues	1. Legal advocate	1. Document from legal advocate
7. Vocational Functioning (e.g., Employment/Education)			
1. Education	1. Obtain GED	1. Contact community agency	1. Bring attendance record
2. Employment	2. Part-time work	2. Job club once a week	2. Attendance
		2. Identify 5 ads each week	2. Show ads and self-report
8. Social Functioning (e.g., Social Support)			
1. Lack of substance-free peer social interaction	1. Develop social support network	1. NA once a day	1. Self report/house manager
		1. Obtain NA sponsor	1. Phone verification
			1. Track NA attendance
2. Drug-using partners	2. Drug-free relationship	2. Couples therapy	2. Track attendance

Figure 6.2 (Continued)

PROBLEM AREA (PRIORITY RANKING)	GOAL	INTERVENTION	OBJECTIVE MEASURE
3. HIV substance/sex risk behaviors	3. No risk behaviors	3. HIV risk reduction skills	3. Track attendance
			3. HIV Behavior Quiz
9. Recreational			
1. Lack of recreational activities	1. Engage in regular substance-free activities	1. Attend 3 recreation activities per week	1. Self-report

Patient's Signature   Date

Counselor's Signature   Date

Figure 6.2 (Continued)

3. Medical problems: Felicia's hepatitis C and anemia

4. Nutrition: may be included in the "food" category in the survival needs section but may also be separate because the patient may have plenty of food, but it lacks adequate nutrients. Thus, the patient would need help selecting different foods for balanced nutrition.

5. Obstetrical treatment: current lack of prenatal care and the need for more regular care

6. Legal assistance: in Felicia's case this would include securing a legal advocate to help her address the warrant for her arrest

7. Vocational functioning: plans to provide education and/or obtain legal employment so that she can become financially independent from family, friends and the government

8. Social functioning: development of a drug-free peer network, potential termination of a relationship with a substance-using male, and tools to reduce HIV risk behaviors

9. Recreational assistance: trying pleasurable activities that are drug-free and participating regularly in them.

Within each of these categories, the specific problem areas are listed separately and are ranked in order of their urgency. After each problem, a goal for resolving it is listed. This goal should be determined and agreed upon by the patient and provider. For example, for the problem of nicotine dependence, it may not be the patient's goal to cease all cigarette use; it may be that at first she will agree only to reduce the number of cigarettes smoked daily. In this case the goal would be specified as "reduction of cigarettes from a pack a day to 10 cigarettes a day."

Once the goal is negotiated, then the intervention that would help the patient to achieve the goal is specified. In the case of her depression symptoms, the patient would receive a referral to be evaluated by a psychiatrist, who would, if appropriate, prescribe an antidepressant medication and also refer her for cognitive-behavioral therapy from a trained counselor.

Once the interventions are determined, there should be methods for measuring progress toward the goals. As often as possible, these methods for determining progress should be objective and quantifiable. In the case of depression, the Beck Depression Inventory (BDI) could be used once a week to assess the presence of depressive symptoms and to determine if their frequency and severity have lessened in comparison to the previous week. There is not an instrument specific to a pregnant population for measuring depressive symptoms, and this is important to note because there is overlap between depressive symptoms and pregnancy symptoms (e.g., sleep changes, weight and appetitive changes, fatigue, etc.), and normal pregnancy symptoms can be misinterpreted as depressive symptoms. Thus, it is important to use an instrument such as the

BDI as a dynamic measure to talk with the patient about what symptoms she is endorsing and why. In other words, the BDI responses can serve as a basis for an interview with the patient in regard to her endorsement of some highly relevant items; as part of that interview, the provider can disentangle which symptoms may be more related to pregnancy and which are related to depression.

As evidenced by the initial treatment plan, pregnant patients being treated for substance use disorders have multiple problems that need to be addressed simultaneously and in an integrated manner. Within each problem area, the provider should prioritize the issues to be addressed and determine whether this order matches the patient's perception of acuity of her own problems. If there is a mismatch between the provider's and the patient's assessment of the priority of treatment needs, they should talk about it and negotiate an agreement. It has been our experience that asking the patient to try it the provider's way first for a set period of time (e.g., 2 weeks) can be helpful; if some specified *intermediate* goals are not attained, then the order of treatment needs can be renegotiated with the patient.

INITIATION OF THE TREATMENT PLAN

Reviewing a long and complex list of issues that a patient has in her life can seem overwhelming for both the patient and provider. When introducing the idea of the treatment plan, there are several key points to keep in mind. First, for a plan to be successful, the patient needs to feel that it is patient-driven and owned by her. Second, the patient needs to be involved in creating the plan as well as all modifications and adjustments in it. Finally, it is important to touch on each issue of concern and have a preliminary plan for addressing each issue. At the same time, it is important not to try to aggressively tackle each issue on the same day or with the same commitment of time and resources.

As discussed in Chapter 13, the provider will want first to address the patient's basic survival needs so that trust and rapport can be established, and so that there is a foundation of basic needs that can be met, before other higher-order issues are tackled. Plans to address housing and food issues are shown in the treatment plan. For example, it may be possible to arrange for a patient to enter and live in a recovery house or other shelter on the same day she enters treatment. For addressing the inadequate food supply, it may be possible to have a goal of obtaining food stamps. As part of this process, it may be that the patient first needs to obtain an identification card in order to apply for or re-establish eligibility for food stamps. Even this goal may need to be broken down into smaller steps, such as gathering the needed papers to provide the patient's address and date of birth and citizenship. In and of itself, these smaller goals of gathering papers and getting the identification card may become part of the treatment plan. Often it is not enough to ask the patient for the necessary papers; rather, a strategy is needed by the provider to assist the patient in planning what information (e.g., papers, birth certificate, etc.) she needs to gather before she goes to the social service center, how she will get to the office, when she will go, if she needs money to pay for the identification card, how she will get this money, and how she will get home. Thinking through the barriers she may encounter and how she will overcome them is a critical step in the treatment plan. Otherwise, the patient may become easily frustrated when any obstacle is encountered, and she may give up and not complete the task.

Once initial concrete plans are made for securing housing and food, then the provider can turn to stabilizing the patient on an opioid agonist medication. Once the patient is stable on her opioid agonist medication, a medication-assisted withdrawal can then occur from benzodiazepines. As described in Chapter 8, it is also suggested that patients are first stabilized in their substance use treatment before assessing for depression or anxiety. Ideally, waiting to assess the patient for these disorders after a two-week period of drug abstinence permits the provider to distinguish substance-induced mood or anxiety disorders from non–substance-induced disorders. Making such a distinction is important to avoid prescribing medication needlessly and exposing a patient and her fetus to the risks. However, some patients do not achieve drug abstinence and could greatly benefit from medication to treat mood disorders. They may be more successful in achieving drug abstinence only after having the mood disorder addressed.

Another issue that could greatly affect treatment for substance use disorders is the patient's legal needs. For example, Felicia has an outstanding warrant for her arrest. She should be assisted in finding legal representation to help her navigate the justice system. She may need to resolve her legal issues before going to the Department of Social Services because she may risk being arrested if the department representative calls the police after searching public files for outstanding arrest warrants.

MONITORING THE TREATMENT PLAN

The treatment plan needs to be considered a dynamic process rather than a static document. Some seemingly important issues on the initial treatment plan may quickly be taken off the list and replaced with other issues because of a change in acuity of the need or the accomplishment of a goal by the patient. It is a good idea to keep a summary of all of the items that are removed from the treatment plan due to the patient meeting her goals. Keeping a chart in the patient's file and showing her the many goals (including the small intermediate ones leading to the larger goal) can serve as a motivator for continued success or a reminder to get the patient back on track. Other items in the treatment plan may need to be revised if the patient is not successful in completing them; a smaller, more manageable intermediate goal that the patient is more likely to reach may be needed before placing the larger goal on the treatment plan.

BREAKING LARGER GOALS INTO SMALLER, MORE MANAGEABLE GOALS

The overall goals of abstinence from heroin and benzodiazepines can by themselves feel overwhelming to patients and need to be broken into smaller goals to provide a "scaffold" to reach this overarching goal. For heroin abstinence, one way to break down this large goal is to first focus on establishing a behavioral contract for 24 or 48 hours of abstinence while the patient is being started on an opioid agonist medication. Once this initial contract has been completed, then a longer period of abstinence can be negotiated in a subsequent contract.

As shown in the example behavioral contract in Figure 6.3, helping patients see their abstinence as a "vacation" from substance use can reduce their resistance to long-term substance use-related behavioral change.

Giving patients direct advice about how to prepare their environment for their lifestyle changes can be beneficial. For example, it may be a good idea to have each overarching treatment goal on a separate page so that there is space on the treatment plan to allow intermediate goals and plans to reach them to be added immediately below the final goal (Fig. 6.4).

Included under the overarching goal of abstinence from heroin can be intermediate goals such as methadone induction, and beside that subgoal can be the objective measure of verification of methadone ingestion. This goal is an "easy" one to meet, and having easy intermediate goals gives patients the opportunity to experience almost-immediate accomplishment. Upon many little successes one can build greater successes. Another intermediate goal under heroin abstinence could be "remove environmental cues to maximize opportunity for sustained abstinence." In the intervention section for that goal can be suggestions such as removing paraphernalia from your house, car, etc.; avoiding places you've used drugs (list places that are safe and not safe to go); avoiding hanging around people who use drugs (list people who are safe and unsafe); and avoiding activities associated with substance use (list activities that you can and can't do—sleep at least 8 hours a night; no commercial sex work). Behavioral items should be verifiable or measurable in some way other than just relying on the patient's self-report.

> We have discussed your treatment, and the importance of entering treatment and starting your vacation from your heroin use.
>
> We know that pregnant women who get treatment for substance use disorders are more likely to have healthier babies and to live healthier lives than women who do not get treatment. For this reason, the treatment team offers the following recommendations to give you the best chance of a healthy life for you and your baby. You have the choice of the 2 options below.
>
> Please circle your selection.
>
> A. Take a vacation from heroin for 24 hours by staying in the in-patient treatment facility.
>
> OR
>
> B. Take a vacation from heroin for 48 hours by staying in the in-patient treatment facility.
>
> I agree to follow the contract for recovery as outlined above. I understand that it is my choice to comply with these recommendations.
>
> _____   _____
> Patient   Date
>
> I agree to reinforce and to honor the efforts the patient makes in complying with this contract. I agree to monitor your progress with this contract.
>
> _____   _____
> Counselor   Date

Figure 6.3 Example of a Behavioral Contract for 24 or 48 Hours of Drug Abstinence

PROBLEM AREA (PRIORITY RANKING)	GOAL	INTERVENTION	OBJECTIVE MEASURE
Psychiatric Treatment: Substance Dependence			
1. Heroin	1. Abstinence	1. Comprehensive treatment	1. Urine sample negative
▶ Intermediate goal: methadone induction		1. Take methadone	1. Verify with pharmacy methadone taken
1a. Benzodiazepine	1a. Abstinence	1a. Medication-assisted withdrawal	1a. Ingestion of less medication
▶ Intermediate goal:	Start benzodiazepine taper	1. Take prescribed benzodiazepine	1. Verify with pharmacy benzo taken as prescribed

Figure 6.4 Example of Goals and Intermediate Goals

MONITORING THE TREATMENT PLAN

The treatment plan needs to be discussed with the patient at every counseling session and on a daily basis when necessary. The successes of meeting the intermediate goals should be carefully tracked and depicted in a tabular or graphic format to show the patient a snapshot of her success in meeting all goals; for each category, the success of meeting intermediate goals can also be shown. The treatment plan should be continually updated with new goals as the old ones are completed. Goals must be appropriate and reachable for each patient's state of recovery. Setting goals that are too high or too difficult to achieve may decrease motivation for drug abstinence or achieving that particular goal, and setting goals that are too easy may also work to reduce motivation.

Preventing Relapse

The best way to prevent relapse is to recognize and address the patient's warning signs before substance use occurs. Observe the patient's clinical presentation at each visit for changes that suggest precursors to relapse. Careful observation and probing questions about the patient's behavior will often reveal what factors (e.g., environmental, personal) need to be in place to support drug abstinence. Typical warning signs of an impending lapse include such things as missing treatment sessions, taking on too many new activities so that attending treatment is difficult, stopping or reducing the number of self-help meetings attended, wanting to use drugs again and not coping with those feelings, going to places where she used substances in the past, hanging out with substance-using friends, and reporting feeling guilty, depressed, overtired, and/or angry.

For example, let's say that Felicia has been attending treatment for her substance use disorder and her prenatal care appointments for the past two months. On Thursday, she mentioned that she was looking forward to the weekend because her favorite boyfriend was being released following a month-long incarceration. The counselor saw this as a warning sign of potential relapse because in the intake interview Felicia had mentioned this was the man with whom she always used drugs. The counselor talked to and role-played with Felicia about the reunion with this boyfriend (e.g., if she must see him, what safe places could she meet him where she would not be temped to use drugs; how she could negotiate protected and drug-free sex with him; etc.). Felicia left her last treatment session on Friday with a concrete plan of where to meet the boyfriend and how to avoid substance use.

On Monday Felicia did not attend treatment, and the counselor called her home that afternoon to express concern and ask why she missed treatment.

Felicia did not answer the phone. On Tuesday, Felicia again did not show up to treatment. The counselor informed the outreach worker, who visited Felicia's home that afternoon and found her on the steps of a neighbor's house with her eyes half-closed, slumped over, with slurred speech when she spoke to the outreach worker. The outreach worker and her safety assistant (outreach workers should always go in pairs, see Chapter 13 for more information on this issue) asked Felicia to come with her in her car so she could be admitted to the inpatient unit. Felicia was at first resistant, saying she needed to pack clothes and could come tomorrow, but the outreach worker pointed out that there is a clothes bank at the center and emphasized how concerned the counselor was about Felicia and the many benefits treatment would provide to her. Felicia returned to treatment with the outreach staff.

Managing Lapse and Relapse

If the patient does lapse (a one-time use of substances) and/or relapse (repeated use of substances), then it is important to understand as much about the episode as possible so that both the counselor and the patient learn from the event and reduce the risk that it will happen again. A functional analysis can be used to understand what events, feelings, and circumstances occurred before the lapse or relapse (the antecedents) and what events, feelings, and circumstances came after the behavior (the consequences). A functional analysis of substance use behavior entails a close look at the circumstances surrounding each episode and what skills and strengths the patient has to use to avoid substance use in the future. An example of a functional analysis can be found in *A Cognitive-Behavioral Approach: Treating Cocaine Addiction* (Carroll, 1998). A functional analysis helps keep the focus off the "why" and onto the "who," "what," "how," "when," and "where" of substance use. The counselor must maintain a neutral tone and body language that is neither punitive nor rewarding of the relapse, allowing the patient and counselor to review what went wrong and to change the treatment plan to minimize continued substance use by the patient.

While substance use of any type can be alarming, the specific drug a patient is using may provide an important clue in determining areas for treatment plan revision. For example, a lapse to opioid use accompanied by withdrawal symptoms may indicate the need for a methadone dose increase. If withdrawal is not indicated and the medication dose is adequate, other factors that might be maintaining her behavior need to be examined (e.g., self-medication to numb the recurrence of intrusive thoughts about rape or other traumatic experiences). If benzodiazepines are being used, the dose of either her methadone or tapering benzodiazepine medication might require adjustment. Although methadone treats only opioid dependence, it may be that the patient is adding additional benzodiazepines to her taper schedule to reduce opioid abstinence symptoms. It may also be that the benzodiazepine taper is too rapid and the rate needs to be slowed. In Felicia's case, while she was living in the inpatient unit "to take a vacation from drug use," as her counselor framed it for her, Felicia had her methadone dose rechecked using both signs and symptoms of withdrawal (these were minimal and then nonexistent), and her plasma level of methadone metabolites was within normal limits. Her counselor performed a functional behavioral analysis with her and, as the counselor suspected, the newly released boyfriend had convinced Felicia to have sex with him after injecting both of them with heroin. Because it was unrealistic for Felicia to leave the boyfriend—she would leave treatment before leaving him—the counselor asked her if the boyfriend would be interested in treatment, and a plan was made to bring him in and facilitate his assessment for methadone treatment the day before Felicia's release from the inpatient unit.

COMPLETION OF THE TREATMENT PLAN

Unfortunately, the length of substance use treatment is often not dictated by the patient's progress or needs for treatment but on the third-party payer's ability to cover the costs of treatment. From the start of the treatment plan, the provider needs to be thinking about how to best prepare and plan for the patient's discharge from the program and where and how she will receive further treatment and care for her ongoing recovery from her substance use disorders, together with gynecological care, other psychiatric care, etc. Unique to treating substance use disorders in pregnant women, the delivery of the baby is an event that can lead to discharge after a few postpartum weeks, given the need for specialized services. Having specific agencies and organizations to which patients can be referred and linked to continue treatment services without interruption is critical for their long-term recovery. Having plans in place for making the transition to a new treatment program and executing these plans, which should include introductions of the patient to the staff at the new care facility, can be critical for ensuring that the patient will follow through with the plan. Often, many of the overall goals in the treatment plan are not fully met, and mechanisms are necessary for ensuring that the patient is referred to services that can help her continue to work toward those overarching goals. The patient should also become an active participant in her discharge and aftercare planning—and, at this point in her treatment process, she should have the tools and skills to handle more of the active establishment of referral connections with less effort from the treatment provider. The treatment plan completion should include a formal recognition that the patient is leaving the program. This could take the form of a certificate accompanied by a graphic summary of all the goals she met during treatment, or a handwritten note from the provider wishing the patient well and summarizing her successes in treatment.

Felicia relapsed to substance use once more after she had completed the initial relapse treatment in the inpatient unit. Her second relapse was triggered by being thrown out of the residence where she was living because she couldn't pay her portion of the rent. While she temporarily moved into a shelter, a move facilitated by her counselor, she used two Xanax pills each day for a week "to deal with the stress and anxiety." This resumption of benzodiazepine use, paired with methadone pharmacotherapy, was especially concerning to the counselor. Again Felicia was admitted to inpatient care to observe and monitor her closely for benzodiazepine withdrawal. The inpatient facility also gave her a place to stay that was drug-free. Her counselor helped her find a long-term residential facility where she could live for the next two years with her child. Two weeks later, while she remained inpatient, Felicia delivered a baby boy, with head circumference, length, and birth weight within normal limits for the delivery at 39 weeks gestational age. Felicia's baby had some signs of withdrawal but these were not severe enough to require medication treatment, and she moved into the long-term residential facility two weeks after delivery, where she could receive her methadone and continue with her job attainment goals through specialized vocational assistance programming.

SUMMARY

Felicia's case illustrates how the initial assessment can be used to develop a comprehensive treatment plan that addresses survival and higher-order life issues. Each patient's multiple problems must be addressed in a systematic and integrated way. The treatment plan should be viewed as a dynamic, ever-changing document that includes both final goals and intermediate goals that the patient can more easily complete as building blocks to reach the overall goals. The goals that are a part of the treatment plan should always be set in discussion with the patient to maximize her belief in herself and her enthusiasm to complete the goals. As soon as the treatment plan is completed and the patient is stabilized, consideration and preparation of the patient for her eventual discharge should be started so that she has the internal and external tools she will need for long-term success.

REFERENCES

Carroll, K. M. (1998). *A cognitive-behavioral approach: treating cocaine addiction.* Therapy Manuals for Drug Abuse: Manual 1, National Institute on Drug Abuse, NIH Publication Number 98–4308.

Jones, H. E., Kaltenbach, K., Coyle, M. G., Heil, S. H., O'Grady, K. E., Arria, A. M., Fischer, G., Stine, S. M., Selby, P., & Martin, P. R . (2009). Re-building lives: Helping women recover from opioid addiction during pregnancy. *Counselor: The Magazine for Addiction Professionals, 10,* 10–19.

Elements of a Model of Care for a Comprehensive Treatment Program for Women with Substance Use Disorders During Pregnancy

7

Helping Patients Stabilize and Withdraw

from Substances

OVERVIEW

This is the first chapter in the third section of the book, and it builds upon the previous chapters that provided information on identification, assessment, and treatment planning followed by implementation of the treatment plan. This third section expands on some of the elements presented in Chapter 6, which gave an overview of treatment planning. In the present chapter we offer an in-depth discussion of the important issues to consider when pregnant patients are being considered as potential candidates for medication-assisted withdrawal from opioids or other substances for which there is need for gradual rather than abrupt cessation of exposure. We must remember that medication-assisted withdrawal is only one component of treatment; it is not a treatment in and of itself (Center for Substance Abuse Treatment [CSAT], 2006).

We define key terms such as medication-assisted withdrawal, also known as detoxification, and discuss why medication-assisted withdrawal may be considered and how it is performed in pregnant patients. We cover the goals of medication-assisted withdrawal and discuss how often it is used for pregnant women. We then present the risks and benefits of medication-assisted withdrawal, followed by its guiding principles. We summarize the specific drugs for which medication-assisted withdrawal may be one component of care. Within each class of drugs, we discuss the common withdrawal signs and symptoms, give examples of tools to measure withdrawal, and explain the medications used to treat withdrawal symptoms specific to that illicit substance. In the latter part of the chapter, we offer guidelines and considerations for managing withdrawal from concomitant substances and ways to facilitate comprehensive treatment services following medication-assisted withdrawal. Finally, we summarize the main themes from the chapter to emphasize learning points.

DEFINITION OF MEDICATION-ASSISTED WITHDRAWAL

Although the term "detoxification" is commonly used in the field of substance use disorder treatment, we will not use it here for two reasons. First, it often carries a stigma, especially for patients who are opioid-dependent and are withdrawing under medical supervision from a prescribed medication such as methadone. Second, detoxification is also defined as a metabolic process in the liver during which the toxic qualities of a poison are reduced by the body. In medication-assisted withdrawal, the patient is stabilized (addressing acute intoxication or withdrawal effects) and then typically is given consecutively smaller doses of a medication that alleviates or suppresses the withdrawal symptoms associated with abrupt cessation of a drug, thereby providing a smoother transition from consistent substance use to a medication-free state (CSAT, 2006; Warner et al., 1997). Examples of the medications used to treat withdrawal signs and symptoms of various classes of substances are discussed below (see "Specific drugs for which medication-assisted withdrawal may be one component of care").

WHY MEDICATION-ASSISTED WITHDRAWAL MAY BE CONSIDERED AND USED IN PREGNANT PATIENTS

The decision to use medication-assisted withdrawal in pregnant patients depends on multiple factors. First, has the patient been prescribed and maintained on the medication for at least several weeks, or has it come from "street" sources? This distinction between withdrawal from a known or unknown source is important as it will influence the starting dose, rate of withdrawal, and type of withdrawal medication used. As will be discussed later in the chapter, there are two classes of substances, opioids and benzodiazepines, from which pregnant patients may be withdrawn following either prescribed maintenance or illegal "street" use. Withdrawing pregnant patients who are stabilized on an opioid agonist should be relatively unusual, as opioid agonist treatment has been found to be effective for pregnant women in treatment for opioid dependence. Other factors to consider in the decision regarding medication-assisted withdrawal include the type of substance she is misusing (or prescribed), the safety and efficacy of the medications available to alleviate the withdrawal she may experience, the patient's desires and expectations for her complete treatment, and the local availability of options and her access to those options. As will be discussed later in this chapter, alcohol and benzodiazepines can pose life-threatening risks if withdrawal is uncontrolled; thus, medication use may be needed to allow safe withdrawal more commonly with these substances than is the case for other substances with less pronounced risks to physical health. Withdrawal from opioids, while not life-threatening for the mother, can produce extreme discomfort, setting the patient up for the risk of relapse and/or termination of treatment. For the embryo and fetus, abrupt withdrawal from exposure to opioids is associated with a risk of spontaneous abortion or miscarriage at worst and at least undue stress. Thus, the need to avoid withdrawal signs and symptoms in pregnant women is repeatedly stated in the clinical literature that discusses this topic (CSAT, 2005; Finnegan, 1991). For the pregnant patient in treatment for opioid dependence, there are two effective medications, methadone and buprenorphine, to treat this disorder. The advantages of methadone maintenance pharmacotherapy, the current "gold standard treatment," over no treatment or medication-assisted withdrawal followed by medication-free treatment include increased rates of treatment retention (Jones et al., 2008), superior relapse prevention, reduced fetal exposure to illicit substance use and other maternal risk behaviors, enhanced compliance with obstetrical care, and enhanced neonatal outcomes (i.e., heavier birth weight; Kaltenbach et al., 1998). Findings in regard to buprenorphine would suggest that it is as efficacious as methadone in terms of maternal outcomes and likely produces superior neonatal outcomes (Jones et al., 2012). In contrast, the use of nicotine replacement treatments for assisting in the cessation of smoking or other tobacco use is controversial (e.g., Einarson, 2006; Morales-Suárez-Varela et al., 2006), and meta-analyses of the literature do not find conclusive support for their efficacy in pregnancy (Coleman et al., 2011). For cocaine and other illicit substances such as methamphetamine, marijuana, inhalants, and hallucinogens, there are no medications for nonpregnant patients; thus, at least a decade of research will be necessary before there are medication options for pregnant women to treat their substance use disorders for a number of substances.

While each pregnant patient is unique and her life circumstances must be carefully considered in the decision to provide medication-assisted withdrawal, there are some occasions in which this procedure may be necessary (Kandall et al., 1999). There are a series of factors to consider when weighing its risks and benefits. These factors would be considered for patients who are either taking prescribed medications (e.g., maintained on methadone or taking benzodiazepines for an anxiety disorder) or misusing medications by "doctor shopping" or "off the street." These factors include:

1. *Strength of the patient's substance-free support network.* The patient may be more likely to succeed in drug abstinence following

medication-assisted withdrawal if her support network includes a number of non–drug-using individuals who are highly supportive of her abstinence—for example, a patient who is the only substance-using person in her family, and her family is highly supportive of her treatment. A patient who has a solid career that she highly values and with which substance use interferes may also be a good candidate for medication-assisted withdrawal.

2. *Strength of comprehensive treatment plan following medication-assisted withdrawal.* Ways to develop and implement a treatment plan were discussed in Chapter 6, and patients may be more likely to remain abstinent if they have a specific treatment plan that includes multiple aspects of continued treatment and they have already started to link to or initiate this continued transition into more formal treatment during the medication-assisted withdrawal process. For example, there have been patients in our program who come to treatment from more than two hours away and are seeking medication-assisted withdrawal so they can qualify for long-term residential treatment in a facility that provides child care, continued abstinence care, job training, and cognitive-behavioral skills. In contrast, other patients have vague plans of treatment continuation that only include "being strong" and "attending Narcotics Anonymous" and who do not yet even have a sponsor for Narcotics Anonymous. For these patients, the likelihood of relapse to substance use is quite high.

3. *Known safety and efficacy of medications to be used for easing withdrawal symptoms.* Any medications used to assist in the medical withdrawal of pregnant patients must have data and good clinical experience to support their use. In general, a long-acting medication such as methadone is preferable to a nonopioid medication (such as clonidine, a central alpha agonist that act in the brain to lower blood pressure) to withdraw pregnant patients from heroin. In the case of benzodiazepines, the provider may want to use the benzodiazepine that the patient has been using and gradually reduce the dose rather than switching the patient to another benzodiazepine, unless the particular benzodiazepine she is using is known to have more deleterious effects on the fetus than another candidate medication.

4. *If medication-assisted withdrawal is not provided, what is the likelihood that the patient will be able to access other care options for her substance use disorder?* In some cases, medication-assisted withdrawal may be the only care option available to the provider and patient to cease the patient's substance use. For example, for patients in rural communities,

medication-assisted withdrawal followed by outpatient counseling may be the only treatment option available.

5. *What is the likelihood that the patient will remove herself from further treatment if withdrawal services are not provided?* Some patients will otherwise refuse treatment entry unless they receive medication-assisted withdrawal. For example, opioid-dependent patients who refuse opioid agonist treatment, like methadone, even after receiving education about some of the myths about the medication are likely candidates for medication-assisted withdrawal. It has been our experience that after starting patients on a methadone-assisted withdrawal, they find that methadone is easily tolerated and not as negative as initially thought. This withdrawal process can provide an extended period during which they may well reconsider agonist medication maintenance.

6. *Are the risks of medication-assisted withdrawal for the mother and her pregnancy greater than no intervention for the disorder?* Usually the risks of gradual medication-assisted withdrawal are not greater than no intervention. One known risk of medication-assisted withdrawal from opioids is the risk for overdose if the patient were to resume opioid use after a period of opioid abstinence. This risk also pertains to benzodiazepines.

To summarize, for opioid- or benzodiazepine-dependent women, the occasions when medication-assisted withdrawal may be useful include when a patient refuses treatment altogether unless she is medication-free at delivery (Martin et al., 1991). For the opioid-dependent pregnant patient, medication-assisted withdrawal may be indicated if agonist maintenance is not available in her community (due to lack of clinic space or the lack of a clinic), or if she needs to take a medication that is incompatible with methadone.

GOALS OF MEDICATION-ASSISTED WITHDRAWAL

The goals of medication-assisted withdrawal include not only eliminating the drug from the patient's body but also maximizing her comfort and therefore the likelihood that she will enter and remain in comprehensive substance use treatment (Polydorou & Kleber, 2008). For patients treated for substance use disorder while pregnant, there is the additional goal of ensuring the safety and health of both mother and fetus. Often, it is neither safe nor practical to have abrupt discontinuation of the substance use.

Thus, using a medication that is of known quantity and quality and appropriately administering it in gradually lower doses will avoid the potentially negative aspects of abrupt cessation of substances such as fetal stress, maternal discomfort, and premature termination of the care services. This goal should be accomplished in a safe, dignified, and humane setting. For example, medication-assisted withdrawal should be conducted in a setting that has staff trained in both psychiatric and obstetrical nursing skills. The setting should be professional and respectful and understanding of the transient discomfort and irritability that patients will feel and express during the process. Certainly an important goal of the process is to maximize the patient's comfort during the drug elimination process. This goal may be accomplished by both nonmedication comfort measures as well as providing adjunct medications that are discussed below.

Medication-assisted withdrawal should be seen as a first step and an initial opportunity to build a therapeutic alliance with the patient and motivate her to enter comprehensive substance use treatment. As discussed in Chapter 6, medication-assisted withdrawal allows the patient to see the benefits of care quickly, and this may motivate her to think seriously about the important and positive life changes that can be made if she continues with treatment. During medication-assisted withdrawal, a comprehensive assessment of multiple areas of life functioning can also be performed (see Chapter 5 for more details on assessment). This assessment will provide a foundation for further treatment planning.

HOW OFTEN MEDICATION-ASSISTED WITHDRAWAL IS USED DURING PREGNANCY

Data from the most recent 2010 National Survey of Substance Abuse Treatment Services reported that 16% of all treatment facilities provide medication-assisted withdrawal and 13% of treatment facilities provide special programs for pregnant/postpartum women. Among women who enter treatment, pregnant women appear to be less likely than nonpregnant women (7% vs. 16%) to enter medication-assisted withdrawal services (Substance Abuse and Mental Health Services Administration, 2011). Pregnant women also appear to be somewhat more likely than nonpregnant women to enter inpatient (35% vs. 20%) and outpatient service settings (78% vs. 74%) (Drug and Alcohol Services Information System, 2004; Substance Abuse and Mental Health Services Administration, 2010). While it is encouraging that pregnant women appear to be less likely to receive medication-assisted withdrawal services than nonpregnant women, these data also suggest that this type of intervention remains one part of the overall treatment continuum; thus, a discussion about why medication-assisted withdrawal may be needed, as well as the other aspects to consider when providing this type of service, is relevant here.

GUIDING PRINCIPLES OF MEDICATION-ASSISTED WITHDRAWAL FROM MISUSED SUBSTANCES FOR PREGNANT PATIENTS

Providers must remember several key principles about medication-assisted withdrawal for pregnant patients. These principles are relevant for opioids, benzodiazepines, and alcohol use disorders.

Medication-assisted withdrawal is not a treatment for a substance use disorder; it represents only one element of a continuum of care. It should never be seen as a standalone treatment; rather, it can serve as an important initial step for patients along the road to recovery and abstinence.

The process of medication-assisted withdrawal has four components: (1) evaluation, (2) stabilization, (3) withdrawal from the substance, and (4) comprehensive treatment. Evaluation should include multiple aspects of the patient's physical, mental, and psychosocial functioning. The severity of withdrawal signs (conditions detected by a health care provider during physical examination of a patient) and symptoms (subjective experiences the patient reports to the health care provider) is assessed repeatedly throughout the day of intake. Stabilization includes the reduction or prevention of withdrawal signs and symptoms, and withdrawal from the substance includes having no medication received and having no withdrawal signs or symptoms. The efficacy of medication-assisted withdrawal should be evaluated based on its ability to produce a physiological state in which the patient is free of her substance of addiction, her withdrawal signs and symptoms are diminished or eliminated, and she enters and remains in a comprehensive or other formal treatment program for substance use disorders.

Medication-assisted withdrawal may be associated with the least risk to the fetus between the second trimester and early third trimester (weeks 14 to 32 of pregnancy). It should not be conducted in either the first trimester, where there is theoretically the greatest risk for spontaneous abortion, or the third trimester, where there is a possibly elevated risk for premature delivery. Regardless of when medication-assisted withdrawal is performed, fetal monitoring should be performed at regular intervals during the tapering. If signs of fetal stress are observed, the withdrawal should be stopped or slowed.

SPECIFIC DRUGS FOR WHICH MEDICATION-ASSISTED WITHDRAWAL MAY BE ONE COMPONENT OF CARE

This section reviews several common classes of substances that are misused by pregnant patients. First discussed are alcohol and benzodiazepines/sedative-hypnotics, either of which can be life-threatening for both mother and the fetus under severe withdrawal conditions. Next discussed are the other types of drugs that are commonly used by pregnant patients with substance use disorders. Within each section, the common withdrawal signs and symptoms are summarized, followed by examples of tools to measure the withdrawal severity. The section ends with an overview of the common types of care used to ease withdrawal from the substance.

ALCOHOL

Signs and Symptoms of Withdrawal

The signs and symptoms of acute alcohol withdrawal typically emerge 6 to 24 hours after the last consumption of alcohol. The signs and symptoms include:

SIMPLER WITHDRAWAL
Signs: loss of appetite, disrupted sleep, restlessness, poor concentration, impaired memory or judgment
Symptoms: anxiety, irritability, agitation, and intense dreams

MORE COMPLEX WITHDRAWAL
Signs: tremors of hands and arms, rapid heartbeat, increased blood pressure, and/or vomiting, increased sensitivity to sound, light and touch, hallucinations (visual, auditory, or tactile), seizures, high fever, delirium and delusions of paranoia
Symptoms: nausea

Measurement instrument to assess withdrawal from alcohol

The Clinical Institute Withdrawal Assessment—Alcohol Revised (CIWA-Ar; Sullivan et al., 1989) has ten items asking about objective (physiological signs) and subjective (e.g., anxiety) aspects of alcohol withdrawal. It takes five minutes to complete. Scores range from 0 to 67. A score of 10 or more indicates clinically significant alcohol withdrawal. The CIWA-Ar requires training to administer and is repeatedly administered during the day (e.g., at each nursing shift).

There are no instruments designed specifically to measure alcohol withdrawal in pregnant women.

Easing Withdrawal

Women undergoing withdrawal from alcohol should receive medication to stabilize them and mitigate any withdrawal symptoms and then should be slowly weaned from the medication in a monitored and supportive health care environment. Protocols for using medications to safely withdraw pregnant patients from alcohol have been described (CSAT, 2006) and will not be reviewed here. In general, benzodiazepines given short term remain the medication of choice for addressing alcohol withdrawal. Weaning the patient from the medication should not be done until all signs and symptoms of withdrawal are mitigated. Nutritional and vitamin supplements should be considered for supportive care (e.g., vitamin B12, iron, etc.) but may not be appropriate for all patients.

BENZODIAZEPINES AND SEDATIVE-HYPNOTICS

Signs and Symptoms of Withdrawal

The onset of withdrawal from short-acting benzodiazepines (e.g., zaleplon [Sonata, Starnoc], zolpidem [Ambien]) often presents early, usually within 24 to 48 hours (British National Formulary, 2009). For benzodiazepines with a long half-life (e.g., flurazepam [Dalmane, Dalmadorm]), the onset of withdrawal may be delayed for up to 3 weeks. The acute benzodiazepine withdrawal syndrome generally lasts for about 2 months, but clinically significant withdrawal symptoms may persist for many months. The severity and length of withdrawal are likely determined by various factors including the rate of tapering, the length of use of benzodiazepines, the dosage, and possibly genetic factors (Higgitt et al., 1985). Withdrawal signs and symptoms from low-dose dependence typically last 6 to 12 months and gradually improve over that period.

Benzodiazepine Withdrawal

SIMPLER WITHDRAWAL

Signs: tremor, muscle twitching, dilated and brisk pupils, headaches, visual disturbance, vomiting/diarrhea

Symptoms: aches and pains, muscle stiffness, dizziness, nausea, agitation, anxiety, panic attacks, depression, irritability, insomnia, perceptual disturbances

More Complex Withdrawal

Signs: grand mal tonic-clonic seizures, delirium, clouding of consciousness, paranoid ideations/delusions, visual and auditory hallucinations, suicidal thoughts

Symptoms: no additional symptoms beyond what were described above for simpler withdrawal

Measurement Instrument to Assess Withdrawal

The Clinical Institute Withdrawal Assessment—Benzodiazepines (CIWA-B; Busto et al., 1986) is used to assess withdrawal from benzodiazepines. This instrument has 20 items, with each item having a scale ranging from 0 to 4. Some questions are rated by the observer and others by the patient. It takes 10 minutes to complete. Scores range from 0 to 80. A score of 10 or more may represent clinically significant withdrawal. The CIWA-B requires training to administer and is repeatedly administered over the course of the day and over the duration of the medication-assisted withdrawal. There are no instruments designed specifically to measure benzodiazepine withdrawal in pregnant women.

Easing Withdrawal

The typical approach to managing benzodiazepine withdrawal is to transfer the pregnant patient to a long-acting benzodiazepine (the most commonly used medication is diazepam [Valium]) and to gradually reduce the dose, with the goal of being substance- and medication-free by the time of delivery (NSW Department of Health, 2006). While this is a laudable goal, tapers from benzodiazepines may take several weeks if not months. Depending on how far advanced the pregnancy is at the time of medication-assisted withdrawal, it may not be possible to taper the medication within the limited time between treatment entry and delivery. In addition to using a medication to ease withdrawal, cognitive and behavioral approaches may ease the patient into a drug-free state.

STIMULANTS, INCLUDING AMPHETAMINES, COCAINE, AND METHAMPHETAMINE

Signs and Symptoms of Withdrawal

The signs and symptoms of withdrawal from cocaine and other stimulants differ greatly from those seen with alcohol, benzodiazepines, and opioids. In contrast to alcohol, benzodiazepines, and opioids, which require assertive treatment for withdrawal, stimulants have less pronounced or outward signs of withdrawal requiring medical intervention or treatment (American Psychiatric Association, 2000). The onset of signs and symptoms of withdrawal from stimulants typically occurs shortly after discontinuation of substance use. The symptoms can abate within 3 to 5 days but may persist for a month (Coffey et al., 2000).

> *Signs:* hypersomnia, lethargy, sudden angry outburst, increased appetite, rapid heartbeat, sleeping too much, sleeping too little, anhedonia
>
> *Symptoms:* fatigue, agitation, depression, anxiety, hyperphagia, hypophagia, carbohydrate craving, cocaine craving intensity, cocaine craving frequency, tension, problems with attention, paranoid suicidal ideation. The most clinically concerning symptom is severe depression, potentially leading to suicidal ideas and attempts.

Measurement Instrument to Assess Withdrawal

Cocaine Selective Severity Assessment (CSSA; Kampman et al., 1998) is a validated instrument that takes 10 minutes to complete. Each of the 18 items on the CSSA is rated on a 0-to-7 scale. The total score is derived by summing the individual items and ranges from 0 to 126. Items that receive the highest score on the CSSA are consistent with criteria for cocaine withdrawal identified in DSM-IV; these include depressed mood, lethargy, increased sleep, increased appetite, and irritability. CSSA scores are specific to cocaine withdrawal; patients withdrawing only from alcohol or opioids do not score high on the CSSA. CSSA scores tend to be higher in patients with more severe cocaine dependence, and scores tend to decline in patients who maintain abstinence (Kampman et al., 1998). There are no known validated tools designed specifically to assess stimulant withdrawal in pregnant patients.

Easing withdrawal

Because there are no medications with empirically tested efficacy to treat stimulant withdrawal, nonpharmacological care is the first line of treatment. Staff trained in nonconfrontational approaches can play an important role in moderating the withdrawal process by using those techniques to avoid escalating irritable, paranoid, and/or agitated patients. To address more severe anxiety or restlessness, hydroxyzine (Vistaril) is a common medication provided to pregnant patients. Diphenhydramine hydrochloride (Benadryl), an antihistamine, is also typically given for restlessness. (Either of these medications may cause dizziness or drowsiness.) During the withdrawal process and during comprehensive treatment, the patient needs to be closely monitored for signs of depression and suicide risk.

OPIOIDS

Signs and Symptoms of Withdrawal

While opioids as a class of drugs generally produce similar withdrawal signs and symptoms, the timing and expression of these signs and symptoms depend on the individual patient. The onset of withdrawal depends in part on the type of opioid used—for example, short-acting opioids such as heroin can result in withdrawal onset 8 to 12 hours after the last administration and may last 3 to 5 days. Withdrawal from longer-acting opioids such as methadone can take 2 to 3 days to be expressed, and symptoms can last up to 3 weeks (Jasinski & Preston, 1995).

> *Signs:* fast heartbeat, high blood pressure, high body temperature, loss of or disrupted sleep, enlarged pupils, abnormally heightened reflexes, sweating, goose bumps, increased breathing, watery eyes, runny nose, yawning, muscle spasm or twitches, vomiting, diarrhea
> *Symptoms:* abdominal cramps, nausea, bone/muscle pains or aches, anxiety

Measurement Instruments to Assess Withdrawal

The Subjective Opiate Withdrawal Scale (SOWS; Handelsman et al., 1987) has 16 items, each rated on a scale of 0 to 4. The SOWS takes 10 minutes to complete; the higher the score, the more severe the withdrawal.

In the Objective Opiate Withdrawal Scale (OOWS; Handelsman et al., 1987), a rater observes the patient for approximately 10 minutes and indicates the presence or absence of 13 items indicating withdrawal. Scores range from 0 to 13, with higher scores indicating more severe withdrawal.

The Clinical Opiate Withdrawal Scale (COWS; Wesson & Ling, 2003) comprises 11 items (1 purely subjective symptom item, 6 objective sign items, and 4 items that include subjective and objective components). Item scoring options vary depending on the item; a higher score on the item indicates more severity. The scores of the items are summed to produce a total score. The higher the total score, the more severe the withdrawal. The COWS has been validated for nonpregnant patients in opioid withdrawal (Tompkins et al., 2009).

The original Clinical Institute Narcotic Assessment (CINA; Peachey & Lei, 1988) comprised 13 items (1 purely subjective symptom item, 7 purely objective sign items, and 5 items that included subjective and objective components). The revised version (Center for Substance Abuse Treatment, 2004; Tompkins et al., 2009) currently in use omits the heart rate and blood pressure items, yielding a scale of 11 items. Item scoring options vary depending on the item; a higher score indicates more severity. The scores of the items are summed to produce a total score. The higher the total score, the more severe the withdrawal.

Research on induction procedures for methadone and buprenorphine patients found that withdrawal symptoms, as measured by the CINA, were not pronounced in either group. Within this low-level withdrawal, buprenorphine-inducted patients showed higher mean peak CINA scores and a steeper trajectory of withdrawal symptoms than did methadone-inducted patients (Holbrook et al., 2012).

With any instrument, clear definitions of items must be provided to patients and staff. Having repeated staff training on how to operationalize the definitions of the withdrawal signs will help maintain consistency in observations over time and with changing staff.

Like the instruments to quantify the withdrawal severity of other substances, there are no known measures intended to assess opioid withdrawal in pregnant women.

Easing Withdrawal

For pregnant patients, methadone is the medication of choice to use as a part of the medical withdrawal process. While specific withdrawal regimens have been provided (CSAT, 2006), data have been published on the relative safety and efficacy of a 7-day methadone withdrawal process in patients who were dependent on heroin and not maintained on methadone prior to withdrawal.

A methadone-assisted withdrawal program that began with methadone 40 mg (all patients received 30 mg and an additional 10 mg was available on the first day) and tapered to 30 mg, 25 mg, 20 mg, 15 mg, 10 mg, and 5 mg per day on days 1 to 7 was found to retain patients in comprehensive substance use treatment significantly longer than a 3-day methadone-assisted withdrawal program (Jones et al., 2008).

Pregnant patients may need concomitant medications to address the withdrawal discomfort that the dose of methadone alone cannot suppress. However, before providing ancillary medications, it may be necessary to consider if the methadone dose is too low. Antacids (e.g., Tums) can be given for indigestion, although they may cause either diarrhea or constipation. For constipation, the first recommendation is to drink water, about three quarts a day, and eat fiber-rich foods. If these dietary changes are not sufficient, docusate sodium (Colace) or milk of magnesia (e.g., Phillips Milk of Magnesia) can be given. Side effects of these medications may include cramping and nausea. To address anxiety or restlessness, as noted above, Vistaril is a common medication provided to pregnant patients, and Benadryl is also typically given for restlessness (either may cause dizziness or drowsiness). Clonidine (Catapres) has also been given to reduce other signs and feelings of withdrawal. Side effects of clonidine may include constipation, nausea, dry mouth, low blood pressure, dizziness, gas, tiredness, or drowsiness. Loperamide (Imodium A-D) may be given for diarrhea. Side effects may include constipation, nausea, gas, and indigestion.

MARIJUANA

Signs and Symptoms of Withdrawal

Marijuana withdrawal typically has an onset of 24 hours after cessation of use.

> *Signs*: restlessness, sleep disturbance, change in eating, tremor, sweating, rapid heartbeat, gastrointestinal disturbance, vomiting, diarrhea
> *Symptoms*: anxiety, irritability, nausea

Measurement Instrument to Assess Withdrawal

The Withdrawal Discomfort Score (WDS; Budney et al., 1999) assesses withdrawal severity by totaling scores from nine items previously reported as common symptoms of withdrawal for *both* cannabis and tobacco: aggression, anger, appetite change (decreased for cannabis, increased for tobacco), depressed mood, irritability, anxiety/nervousness, restlessness, sleep difficulty, and strange dreams (American Psychiatric Association, 2000). The WDS has shown good internal consistency (internal consistency α = .89) in nonpregnant samples (Budney et al., 1999). This withdrawal measure, like the other instruments discussed in this chapter, has not been validated in pregnant patients.

Easing Withdrawal

There are no medications or marijuana-specific withdrawal treatments.

NICOTINE

Signs and Symptoms of Withdrawal

Nicotine withdrawal typically is experienced starting a few hours to 24 hours after the last use of tobacco.

Signs: decreased heart rate, increased eating or weight gain, restlessness, difficulty concentrating, difficulty sleeping
Symptoms: increased appetite, anxiety, irritability, frustration or anger, dysphoric or depressed mood

Nicotine withdrawal signs and symptoms can be confused with other psychiatric conditions (e.g., depression, anxiety).

Measurement Instrument to Assess Withdrawal

The Minnesota Withdrawal Scale–Revised (developed by Hughes & Hatsukami, 2008) is available at http://www.uvm.edu/~hbpl/minnesota/2008/Instructions. pdf. The patient-rating version has 15 items, and the patient responds to each item using a 4-point scale. There is also an observer scale that has five items. These scales have not been validated in pregnant women.

Easing Withdrawal

Smoking cessation is extremely difficult, and it may be even more difficult during pregnancy due to the increased rate of metabolism of nicotine and cotinine (the nicotine metabolite), with increased clearance from the body of 60% and 140%, respectively. This faster clearance of nicotine from the pregnant woman's body means she may need to smoke more cigarettes to achieve the same effect as when she was not pregnant (Dempsey et al., 2002).

In terms of medication options, nicotine replacement is the best-known and most-studied choice in pregnant women. Nicotine replacement can be delivered in various forms, including a patch, lozenge, gum, inhaler, and nasal spray. Because the nicotine patch has been available for years, it is the cessation method used in most pregnancy studies. Studies conducted using nicotine replacement generally have not been very successful, possibly because the increased clearance during pregnancy results in participants not receiving high enough doses of nicotine, resulting in poor compliance (Hotham et al., 2006; Selby et al., 2001). The largest study using nicotine replacement therapy in pregnant women showed no differences between its use and placebo (Schroeder et al., 2002).

Two other pharmacotherapies, the smoking cessation agent varenicline and the antidepressant bupropion, have been successfully used with nonpregnant patients. However, there is insufficient information on the adverse effects associated with either medication to recommend their use to aid in smoking cessation in pregnant women (Cressman et al., 2012), and there are some data suggesting that buproprion may be associated with congenital heart defects (Alwan et al., 2010). Finally, no information is available regarding the safety of breastfeeding for the neonate while the mother is maintained on either varenicline or buproprion.

CHALLENGE OF TREATING WITHDRAWAL FROM MULTIPLE SUBSTANCES

The prevalent comorbid misuse of alcohol, benzodiazepines, and/or opioids in any combination raises alarm for several reasons. First, both alcohol and benzodiazepines have the potential to augment the central nervous system depressant effects together and with methadone and buprenorphine (e.g., Lintzeris et al., 2006, 2007). As such, these substances are considered as risk factors for a lethal outcome in combination with each other or in combination with opioids. Combinations of alcohol, benzodiazepines, and opioids can also increase the risk of compromised cognitive or motor performance as well as poor psychosocial functioning and treatment response (e.g., Clark et al., 2006).

Addressing combinations of alcohol and/or benzodiazepine and/or opioid misuse is especially challenging in the pregnant patient. Very little is known about the effects of the combination of opioids with alcohol and/or benzodiazepines on the mother, the fetus, or the neonate. Opioid-dependent patients who are diagnosed as alcohol-dependent must be detoxified from alcohol immediately, because alcohol withdrawal is potentially more dangerous than opioid or benzodiazepine withdrawal to both mother and fetus. Detoxification can be accomplished using an evidence-based withdrawal protocol for alcohol dependence and a symptom-triggered approach to diazepam dosing using the CIWA-Ar scale (Sullivan et al., 1989).

The need for a medication taper to avoid complicating benzodiazepine withdrawal in the opioid-dependent patient would also be performed using diazepam to suppress withdrawal symptoms (measured by the CIWA-B; Busto et al., 1986) and then subsequently reducing the dose over time. However, it is suggested that stabilizing opioid dependence should be accomplished before initiating the benzodiazepine taper because opioid dependence is more easily and more quickly treated and thus much easier to manage. Moreover, there tend to be more risky behaviors surrounding opioid use relative to benzodiazepine use in some but not all cases.

OTHER MEDICAL CONSIDERATIONS THAT MAY EXACERBATE OR OVERLAP WITH WITHDRAWAL SIGNS AND SYMPTOMS

Many patients with substance use disorders have abnormal glucose levels. An abnormally high or low blood sugar level can be confused with the signs and symptoms of withdrawal. Thus, a check of the blood glucose level is important, especially in pregnant patients. Hypoglycemia (low blood sugar level) can lead to mood changes, and these mood changes can be exacerbated in patients with substance use disorders. When blood glucose levels are below normal levels, patients may feel depressed, anxious, and moody and/or crave drugs (CSAT, 2006).

EDUCATING PATIENTS ON THE WITHDRAWAL PROCESS

Before any medication-assisted withdrawal process begins, it is important to educate the patient, and with her permission the family or supportive others in her life, about what will happen during and immediately after this intervention. Any information given verbally should also be provided in writing using a low-grade reading level and short, simple, bulleted-style handouts. Informing the patient that, typically, withdrawal effects from a substance are the opposite effects that the drug provides will help her understand what to expect and reduce anxiety. Providing the patient with some behavioral tools that she can use to counteract some of the discomfort without relapsing to drugs may also be helpful in bolstering her ability to adhere to the withdrawal process. Staff should be realistic about the discomfort that she might feel and should assure her that everything that can be done to maximize her tolerance of the process will be provided. Finally, ensuring that the patient understands that the medication-assisted withdrawal process is only the first step in a complete treatment process is essential to ensuring that she continues in comprehensive care.

LINKAGE TO COMPREHENSIVE TREATMENT

As soon as the patient is stabilized, the focus should turn to comprehensive treatment. For patients who are to receive a medication-assisted withdrawal, a plan for comprehensive care needs to be in place before the withdrawal starts. While specific tools regarding how to enhance patient response to linkage referrals and comprehensive treatment are discussed in Chapter 13, it is worth noting here that preparation for continued treatment should focus on minimizing as many external and internal barriers as possible—for example, helping the patient navigate complicated insurance systems to receive care, and using Motivational Interviewing techniques to bolster the patient's motivation to continue treatment. Patients are more likely to initiate and stay in treatment if they believe the services will help them with specific life problems (Fioretine et al., 1999). The importance of linkage to formal treatment that addresses the multiple and complex challenges patients frequently face in their lives cannot be overstated. Substance use disorders that are treated during pregnancy almost always start before pregnancy, and this complicated illness is best treated with an equally comprehensive treatment.

SUMMARY

Medication-assisted withdrawal should not be considered a treatment for substance abuse when given in isolation; however, it can be an engaging first step for pregnant patients not already in treatment to promote entry into comprehensive treatment. Aspects of medication-assisted withdrawal include stabilization from acute intoxication or withdrawal, continued suppression of withdrawal signs and symptoms with consecutively lower doses of medication, and achievement of a drug-free state. For patients withdrawing from a prescribed medication such as methadone or benzodiazepines, the process must be completed without uncomfortable withdrawal signs and symptoms; the process must be halted if it becomes intolerable. Medication-assisted withdrawal from any substance should be conducted only if (1) the patient is well informed, (2) the medication used is appropriate, (3) there is close fetal and maternal monitoring, and (4) the process is followed by linkage to comprehensive treatment.

REFERENCES

Alwan, S., Reefhuis, J., Botto, L. D., Rasmussen, S. A., Correa, A., & Friedman, J. M. (2010); National Birth Defects Prevention Study. Maternal use of bupropion and risk for congenital heart defects. *American Journal of Obstetrics and Gynecology, 203*(1), 52.e1–6.

American Psychiatric Association. (2000). *Diagnostic and statistical manual of mental disorders* (4th ed. Text Revision). Washington, DC: American Psychiatric Association.

British National Formulary. (2009). *Hypnotics and anxiolytics.* British National Formulary.

Budney, A. J., Novy, P. L., & Hughes, J. R. (1999). Marijuana withdrawal among adults seeking treatment for marijuana dependence. *Addiction, 94*(9), 1311–1322.

Busto, U., Sellers, E. M., Naranjo, C. A., Cappell, H., Sanchez-Craig, M., & Sykora, K. (1986). Withdrawal reaction after long-term therapeutic use of benzodiazepines. *New England Journal of Medicine, 315,* 854–859.

Center for Substance Abuse Treatment. (2004). *Clinical guidelines for the use of buprenorphine in the treatment of opioid addiction.* Treatment Improvement Protocol (TIP) Series 40. DHHS Publication No. (SMA) 04-3939. Rockville, MD: Substance Abuse and Mental Health Services Administration.

Center for Substance Abuse Treatment. (2005). *Medication-assisted treatment for opioid addiction in opioid treatment programs.* Treatment Improvement Protocol (TIP) Series 43. DHHS Publication No. (SMA) 05-4048. Rockville, MD: Substance Abuse and Mental Health Services Administration.

Center for Substance Abuse Treatment. (2006). *Detoxification and substance abuse treatment.* Treatment Improvement Protocol (TIP) Series 45. DHHS Publication No. (SMA) 06-4131. Rockville, MD: Substance Abuse and Mental Health Services Administration.

Clark, N. C., Dietze, P., Lenne, M. G., & Redman, J. R. (2006). Effect of opioid substitution therapy on alcohol metabolism. *Journal of Substance Abuse Treatment, 30*(3), 191–196.

Coffey, S. F., Dansky, B. S., Carrigan, M. H., & Brady, K. T. (2000). Acute and protracted cocaine abstinence in an outpatient population: a prospective study of mood, sleep and withdrawal symptoms. *Drug and Alcohol Dependence, 59*(3), 277–286.

Coleman, T., Chamberlain, C., Cooper, S., & Leonardi-Bee, J. (2011). Efficacy and safety of nicotine replacement therapy for smoking cessation in pregnancy: Systematic review and meta-analysis. *Addiction, 106*(1), 52–61.

Cressman, A. M., Pupco, A., Kim, E., Koren, G., & Bozzo, P. (2012). Smoking cessation therapy during pregnancy. *Canadian Family Physician, 8*(5), 525–527.

Dempsey, D., Jacob, P. 3rd, & Benowitz, N. L. (2002). Accelerated metabolism of nicotine and cotinine in pregnant smokers. *Journal of Pharmacology and Experimental Therapeutics, 301,* 594–598.

Drug and Alcohol Services Information System (DASIS) (2004). *Pregnant women in substance abuse treatment: 2002.* Office of Applied Studies, SAMHSA; Synectics for Management Decisions, Inc., Arlington, VA; RTI International, Research Triangle Park, NC.

Einarson, A. (2006). Smoking during pregnancy versus no smoking and using nicotine replacement therapies (NRT). *Journal of Fetal Alcohol Syndrome International, 4*(4), 1–2.

Finnegan, L. P. (1991). Treatment issues for opioid-dependent women during the perinatal period. *Journal of Psychoactive Drugs, 23*(2), 191–201.

Fiorentine, R., Nakashima, J., & Anglin, M. D. (1999). Client engagement in drug treatment. *Journal of Substance Abuse Treatment, 17*(3), 199–206.

Handelsman, L., Cochrane, K. J., Aronson, M. J., Ness, R., Rubinstein, K. J., & Kanof, P. D. (1987). Two new rating scales for opiate withdrawal. *American Journal of Drug and Alcohol Abuse, 13*(3), 293–308.

Higgitt, A. C., Lader, M. H., & Fonagy, P. (1985). Clinical management of benzodiazepine dependence. *British Medical Journal (Clinical Research Edition), 291,* 688–690.

Holbrook, A. M., Jones, H. E., Heil, S. H., Martin, P. R., Stine, S. M., Fischer, G., Coyle, M. G., & Kaltenbach, K. (2012, in preparation). Induction of pregnant women onto opioid-agonist medication: an analysis of withdrawal symptoms and study retention.

Hotham, E. D., Gilbert, A. L., & Atkinson, E. R. (2006). A randomised-controlled pilot study using nicotine patches with pregnant women. *Addictive Behaviors, 31*(4), 641–648.

Hughes, J. R., & Hatsukami, D. (2008). Instructions for use of the Minnesota Withdrawal Scale-Revised. Available online: http://www.uvm.edu/~hbpl/minnesota/2008/Instructions.pdf (accessed August 16, 2009).

Jasinski, D. R., & Preston, K. L. (1995). Laboratory studies of buprenorphine in opioid abusers. In A. Cowan & J. W. Lewis (Eds.), *Buprenorphine: Combatting drug abuse with a unique opioid* (pp. 189–211). New York: Wiley-Liss.

Jones, H. E., Arria, A. M., Baewert, A., Heil, S. H., Kaltenbach, K., Martin, P. R., Coyle, M. G., Selby, P., Stine, S. M., & Fischer, G. (2012). Buprenorphine treatment of opioid-dependent pregnant women: A comprehensive review. *Addiction, 107*(Suppl. 1), 5–27.

Jones, H. E., O'Grady, K. E., Malfi, D., & Tuten, M. (2008). Methadone maintenance vs. methadone taper during pregnancy: maternal and neonatal outcomes. *American Journal on Addictions, 17*(5), 372–386.

Kaltenbach, K., Berghella, V., & Finnegan, L. (1998). Opioid dependence during pregnancy. Effects and management. *Obstetrics & Gynecology Clinics of North America, 25*(1), 139–151.

Kampman, K. M., Volpicelli, J., McGinnis, D., Alterman, A. I., Weinrieb, R., D'Angelo, L., & Epperson, L. (1998). Reliability and validity of the cocaine selective severity assessment. *Addictive Behaviors, 23*, 449–461.

Kandall, S. R., Doberczak, T. M., Jantunen, M., & Stein, J. (1999). The methadone-maintained pregnancy. *Journal of Perinatology, 26*, 173–183.

Lintzeris, N., Mitchell, T. B., Bond, A., Nestor, L., & Strang, J. (2006). Interactions on mixing diazepam with methadone or buprenorphine in maintenance patients. *Journal of Clinical Psychopharmacology, 26*, 274–283.

Lintzeris, N., Mitchell, T. B., Bond, A.J., Nestor, L., & Strang, J . (2007). Pharmacodynamics of diazepam co-administered with methadone or buprenorphine under high-dose conditions in opioid-dependent patients. *Drug and Alcohol Dependence, 91*, 187–194.

Martin, J., Payte, J. T., & Zweben, J. E. (1991). Methadone maintenance treatment: a primer for physicians. *Journal of Psychoactive Drugs, 23*(2), 165–176.

Morales-Suarez-Varela, M. M., Bille, C., Christensen, K., & Olsen, J. (2006). Smoking habits, nicotine use, and congenital malformations. *Obstetrics and Gynecology. 107*(1), 51–57.

NSW Department of Health. (2006, March). National Clinical Guidelines for the Management of Drug Use During Pregnancy, *Birth and the Early Development Years of the Newborn.* http://www.health.nsw.gov.au/pubs/2006/pdf/ncg_druguse.pdf. (accessed October 27, 2012).

Peachey, J. E., & Lei, H. (1988). Assessment of opioid dependence with naloxone. *British Journal of Addictions, 83*, 193–201.

Polydorou, S., & Kleber, H. (2008). Chapter 19: Detoxification of Opioids. In M. Galanter & H. Kleber (Eds.), *American Psychiatric Publishing textbook of substance abuse treatment* (pp. 265–288). Arlington, VA: American Psychiatric Publishing.

Schroeder, D. R., Ogburn, P. L. Jr, Hurt, R. D., Croghan, I. T., Ramin, K. D., Offord, K. P., & Moyer, T. P. (2002). Nicotine patch use in pregnant smokers: smoking abstinence and delivery outcomes. *Journal of Maternal-Fetal and Neonatal Medicine, 11*(2), 100–107.

Selby, P., Hackman, R., Kapur, B., Klein, J., & Koren, G. (2001). Heavily smoking women who cannot quit in pregnancy: evidence of pharmacokinetic predisposition. *British Medical Journal (Clinical Research Edition), 23*(3), 189–191.

Substance Abuse and Mental Health Services Administration. (2010). *National survey of substance abuse treatment services.* Available online: http://www.icpsr.umich.edu/icpsrweb/SAMHDA/studies/32723 (accessed July 29, 2012).

Substance Abuse and Mental Health Services Administration. (2011). *National Survey of Substance Abuse Treatment Services (N-SSATS): 2010. Data on Substance Abuse Treatment Facilities.* DASIS Series S-59, HHS Publication No. (SMA) 11-4665. Rockville, MD: Substance Abuse and Mental Health Services Administration.

Sullivan, J. T., Sykora, K., Schneiderman, J., Naranjo, C. A., & Sellers, E.M. (1989). Assessment of alcohol withdrawal: the revised Clinical Institute Withdrawal Assessment for Alcohol scale (CIWA-Ar). *British Journal of Addiction, 84*(11), 1353–1357.

Tompkins, D. A., Bigelow, G. E., Harrison, J. A., Johnson, R. E., Fudala, P. J., & Strain, E. C. (2009). Concurrent validation of the Clinical Opiate Withdrawal Scale (COWS) and single-item indices against the Clinical Institute Narcotic Assessment (CINA) opioid withdrawal instrument. *Drug Alcohol Dependence, 105*(1–2), 154–159.

Warner, E. A., Kosten, T. R., & O'Connor, P. G. (1997). Pharmacotherapy for opioid and cocaine abuse. *Medical Clinics of North America, 81*, 909–925.

Wesson, D. R., & Ling, W. (2003). The Clinical Opiate Withdrawal Scale (COWS). *Journal of Psychoactive Drugs, 35*, 253–259.

8

Caring for the Dually Diagnosed Patient

OVERVIEW

As first presented in Chapter 5, all pregnant patients with a substance use disorder should be evaluated for any co-occurring psychiatric disorders. These disorders should be treated and systematically monitored. This topic was discussed in Chapter 6 as an intrinsic part of treatment planning. In this chapter we expand upon the discussion of the treatment of substance use disorders in the pregnant patient who also has co-occurring psychiatric diagnoses.

Pregnant patients entering treatment for substance use disorders often present with multiple psychiatric disorders. The treatment of these comorbid psychiatric disorders is complicated by the need to balance the risks and benefits of treatment for the mother's health and well-being with the health of the fetus. These risks and benefits are interrelated and sometimes pose potentially competing interests. In this chapter we first present the prevalence and consequences of the most common psychiatric disorders for which pregnant patients with substance use disorders may also need care during substance use treatment. Next, we present strategies for treating these comorbid disorders and the risk/benefit considerations that are needed for an informed treatment approach to these disorders. Then, we offer practical strategies for facilitating the patient's participation in the treatment of comorbid psychiatric disorders. Finally, the take-home messages of the chapter are summarized.

PREVALENCE OF THE MOST COMMON PSYCHIATRIC DISORDERS

Comparing across studies of pregnant patients, women with substance use disorders have greater rates of depression and anxiety than pregnant patients without such substance use (e.g., Battle et al., 2006; Kessler et al., 1997; Kissin et al., 2001; Martin et al., 2009).

Compared to what is known about depression and anxiety disorders, much less information is available on other comorbid psychiatric disorders among pregnant patients being treated for substance use disorders. In one sample of pregnant patients with substance use disorders, mood disorders were most common, with 46% and 40% of the sample meeting criteria for hypomania and major depression, respectively. Positive screens for anxiety disorders were also common: 43% of the sample met criteria for generalized anxiety disorder and 28% met criteria for panic disorder. Agoraphobia (26%), social phobia/social anxiety (22%), and posttraumatic stress disorder (PTSD; 18%) were also present (Martin et al., 2009). Less common were bulimia (10%) and obsessive-compulsive disorders (5%) (Martin et al., 2009). Among the 1,000+ pregnant substance-dependent women whom we have screened for research at the Center for Addiction and Pregnancy over the past 10 years, we have observed that schizophrenia is relatively rare (current prevalence of 1% to 2%, which is similar to the rate in the general population). It has also been observed that other psychiatric disorders, including bipolar and dysthymia, occur in less than 5% of substance-dependent pregnant patients (e.g., Kissin et al., 2001). Although these prevalence data may be unique to the Center for Addiction and Pregnancy, space limitations preclude a discussion of every type of comorbid psychiatric disorder that a provider may encounter in pregnant patients treated for substance use disorders. As such, we devote the remainder of this chapter to the most common comorbid disorders that a provider may encounter in this population.

MOOD DISORDERS

Types of Mood Disorders

Mood disorders typically diagnosed in pregnant patients with substance use disorders include major depression, bipolar disorder, and dysthymic disorder. Major depression involves a loss of interest or pleasure in the patient's typical daily activities along with other symptoms such as appetite changes, sleep disturbances, loss of energy, and suicidal thoughts. Bipolar disorder includes mania, elevated or expansive mood, irritable mood, and other signs such as rapid speech, restlessness, and increased activity. Dysthymic disorder is characterized by depressive symptoms that occur for most of the day, more days than not, for at least 2 years (American Psychiatric Association, 1995). In adults, up to 75% of individuals with this disorder will develop major depression within 5 years (http://www.mentalhealth.com/dis/p20-md04.html).

Depression During Pregnancy

During pregnancy, depression is one of the most common and yet under-identified and untreated comorbid disorders. This is true for both the general pregnant population and pregnant women with substance use disorders. Depression during pregnancy has been associated with tobacco use, substance use disorders, hypertension, preeclampsia, and gestational diabetes (see Grote et al., 2010, for a summary). In the general population, prevalence rates of depressive symptoms were 8% to 13% during pregnancy (Gavin et al., 2005; Vesga-López et al., 2008) and 7%, 13%, and 12% during the first, second, and third trimesters, respectively (Bennett et al., 2004). Women in poverty are also more likely than middle-class women to experience depression (Grote et al., 2010). If left untreated, mood and other psychiatric disorders are associated with increased pregnancy- and neonatal-related morbidity and mortality (Field et al., 2008; Misri & Kendrick, 2007). Depression in pregnant patients can be difficult to conclusively determine because some symptoms, such as change in appetite, loss of energy, excessive fatigue, sleep disturbances, and change in sex drive, can be expected as part of a normal pregnancy.

Consequences of Co-occurring Depression and Substance Use Disorders in Pregnant Patients

OVERLAP IN DISORDERS

Patients with depression or anxiety are more likely than the general population to smoke tobacco and use mood-altering substances. Depressed pregnant women are more likely than nondepressed pregnant women to use antiemetics, opioid analgesics, and all prescription drugs. In contrast, pregnant women with anxiety are more likely than nonanxious pregnant women to use benzodiazepines (Newport et al., 2012). Further, patients with substance use disorders who become pregnant have a generally higher risk of experiencing depression during pregnancy than the larger population. It is estimated that between 40% and 73% of women with substance use disorders have comorbid depression (Burns et al., 1985; Fitzsimons et al., 2007; Haller et al., 1993; Martin et al., 2009), and among pregnant women with substance use disorders, almost 50% have been found to have postpartum depression at 6 weeks after delivery (Holbrook & Kaltenbach, 2012).

NEGATIVE MATERNAL OUTCOMES ASSOCIATED WITH DEPRESSION

Depression is an important disorder to recognize and treat because it has been associated with negative outcomes of maternal substance use treatment.

Examples of these detrimental outcomes related to depressive symptoms in a sample of pregnant methadone-maintained women include less clinic attendance (Finnegan, 1981) and greater rates of drug-positive urine samples while in treatment (Benningfield et al., 2012; Fitzsimons et al., 2007). Moreover, cocaine-using pregnant women enrolled in substance use treatment were more likely to terminate treatment if they had current mood disorders compared to women who did not have such disorders (Haller et al., 2002), and opioid-dependent pregnant women with symptoms of anxiety were more likely to discontinue treatment compared to opioid-dependent pregnant women who reported neither depression nor anxiety symptoms (Benningfield et al., 2012).

Negative Birth Outcomes Associated with Depression

Depression during pregnancy is also associated with adverse pregnancy outcomes such as premature birth, lower birth weight, and neonatal behavioral effects (Cohen et al., 2004; Diego et al., 2009; Field et al., 2008;Wisner et al., 2000). A recent meta-analysis of depression during pregnancy found that it increases the risk for preterm birth and low birth weight (Grote et al., 2010). Data have repeatedly shown that prenatal depression is associated with more neonatal crying (Diego et al., 2004; Field et al., 2007; Zuckerman et al., 1990), greater newborn inconsolability (Zuckerman et al., 1990) less verified sleep behavior (Diego et al., 2004, 2009), and more activity and movement (Field et al., 2007, 2008). The role that the combination of substance use exposure and depression plays in compromising neonatal and early childhood development is sorely in need of research. The available data from a sample of methadone-maintained patients showed that neonates from mothers with a primary mood disorder diagnosis had longer stays in the neonatal intensive care unit, on average, than did the offspring of those without a current mood disorder (Tuten et al., 2009).

Bipolar disorder and dysthymia are much less common in the pregnant population in treatment for a substance use disorder and thus are beyond the scope of this chapter.

ANXIETY DISORDERS

Types of Anxiety Disorders

Anxiety disorders include phobias, panic disorders, generalized anxiety disorders, obsessive-compulsive disorders, and PTSD. There are three major types of phobias: agoraphobia, social, and simple. Agoraphobia is characterized by fear of being alone in public places where escape may be difficult. Panic attacks can accompany this disorder. A social phobia is an intense fear of and desire to avoid objects or situations. A generalized anxiety disorder is a pattern of constant worry or anxiety over the activities of daily life, without any reasonable cause for the concern. An obsessive-compulsive disorder involves obsessions and/or compulsions that are distressing and interfere with daily functions. PTSD involves the re-experiencing of a psychologically traumatic event though dreams, along with numbing and reduced responsiveness (First et al., 1997). There is literature to support a pregnancy-specific anxiety, a distinct syndrome that includes fears about the baby's health and well-being, the health care experience, survival during pregnancy, and the parenting role. Pregnancy anxiety has been found to reliably predict the timing of delivery, with the greater stress predicting an earlier delivery (Schetter & Tanner, 2012).

Consequences of Anxiety During Pregnancy

In contrast to the conclusive data regarding the detrimental consequences of depression during pregnancy, less consistent data are available for the anxiety disorders. A meta-analytic review (Littleton et al., 2007) showed that anxiety symptoms were not significantly correlated with perinatal outcomes. One important limitation of the research on anxiety disorders during pregnancy is the focus on general anxiety symptoms, which may not be representative of actual diagnosed anxiety disorders in the pregnant population. It is quite possible that only the more severe anxiety disorders are associated with poorer perinatal outcomes.

PTSD
One example of a severe anxiety disorder is PTSD. Significant predictors of trauma exposure have included either a preexisting substance use disorder or a preexisting anxiety disorder. Once a trauma exposure occurs, the strongest predictors of PTSD symptoms were being female and the type of trauma, either physical or sexual in nature (Perkonigg et al., 2000). These prospective findings have been supported by other cross-sectional studies showing that PTSD is more common among women than men and that women tend to have different types of precipitating traumas and higher rates of comorbid panic disorder and agoraphobia than do men (Nemeroff et al., 2006).

PTSD has been reported to be associated with adverse pregnancy outcomes. Women with PTSD have a greater likelihood than women without a psychiatric diagnosis for ectopic pregnancy (pregnancy outside the uterus), spontaneous abortion, premature contractions, and excessive fetal growth (Seng et al., 2001). PTSD is also strongly associated with interpersonal violence, depression, and low birth weight (Rosen et al., 2007). PTSD subsequent to child abuse trauma exposure has been found to be strongly associated with adverse outcomes, including lower gestational age at delivery and low birth weight (Seng et al., 2011). Because depression, violence, trauma, and substance use can all affect maternal health and birth outcomes in substance-dependent women, they must be treated in a concurrent and integrated manner.

In pregnant patients treated for substance use disorders, the lifetime diagnosis rate of PTSD is 19% (Moylan et al., 2001) and the current screening diagnosis rate is 18% (Martin et al., 2009). Among substance-dependent pregnant patients, on average, patients with a lifetime diagnosis of PTSD reported a greater need for psychiatric treatment, were more likely have previously attempted suicide, and had a greater number of previous substance use treatments than participants without PTSD (Moylan et al., 2001). On a positive note, among pregnant patients with a substance use disorder, patients with comorbid anxiety disorders attended, on average, more days of substance use treatment than did patients with comorbid mood disorder or no other comorbid disorder (Fitzsimons et al., 2007).

To the best of our knowledge, no studies have examined the relationship between PTSD and substance use disorders and maternal and neonatal outcomes.

DETERMINING THE TEMPORAL RELATIONSHIP BETWEEN SUBSTANCE USE AND THE COMORBID PSYCHIATRIC SYMPTOMS

Classifying Axis I psychiatric disorders as substance-induced or independent disorders can be helpful in guiding treatment of both disorders. Emphasizing the temporal relationship between increases or reductions in substance use and the psychiatric symptoms being evaluated can aid in an understanding of the need either to concurrently treat the substance use disorder and other Axis I disorder or to treat only the substance use disorder (King & Brooner, 1999). If the comorbid disorder is substance-induced, the symptoms will be time-limited and will abate if appropriate substance use treatment is first provided to the patient and she remains abstinent from drugs. Knowing whether a patient treated for substance use disorders experienced symptoms during weeks or months of continuous abstinence may suggest the independence of the comorbid psychiatric disorder (King & Brooner, 1999). However, many pregnant patients typically lack any substantial time of drug abstinence to be able to properly evaluate this issue.

TREATMENT OF COMORBID PSYCHIATRIC DISORDERS DURING PREGNANCY

As described earlier in the chapter, patients treated for substance use disorders during pregnancy may have suboptimal substance use treatment and pregnancy outcomes; thus, the identification of comorbid psychiatric disorders can provide useful markers for patients at risk for poor response to traditional substance use disorder treatment. Patients may need specialized treatment or additional treatment resources to improve their adherence to treatment goals and improve functioning in multiple life areas that could be impaired by the comorbid disorders. Currently, the approaches to treating Axis I disorders in patients who also have substance use disorders include both behavioral and medication options.

Behavioral Treatment Approaches

BEHAVIORAL TREATMENTS FOR DEPRESSION

Recent efforts to treat depression and comorbid substance use disorders have focused on integrated treatments (e.g., Weiss, 2004). As described in Chapter 2, cognitive-behavioral therapies are among the most powerful behavioral treatments for depression and also have proven efficacy for substance use disorders. Cognitive-behavioral therapy (CBT) focuses on the relationship between thoughts, emotions, and behaviors and teaches the patient skills for managing these relationships. Several studies have shown that in the treatment of depression, the success rate of CBT is no different from that of medication (Hollon et al., 1992); however, these effects have not been examined in pregnant patients or pregnant patients with substance use disorders.

BEHAVIORAL TREATMENTS FOR ANXIETY

In nonpregnant patients, generalized anxiety disorder, panic disorder, or other anxiety disorders are typically treated with specific CBT combined with antidepressant or buspirone (Buspar) treatment. It has been suggested that even if specialized care is not available, medication plus supportive counseling can help patients improve (King et al., 1999). While there are no clinical studies of Buspar in pregnant patients with substance use disorders, it is classified in U.S. Food and Drug Administration (FDA) pregnancy category B (no evidence of risk of harm to humans during pregnancy; see Table 8.1 for more information) due to the lack of teratogenic evidence in animals and humans.

Medication Treatment Approaches

In the past decade, tremendous progress has been made in developing and approving medications to treat a variety of diseases and disorders that affect pregnant women. Since almost no clinical trials include pregnant women, the vast majority of medications are classified as FDA category C (i.e., no information regarding their use in pregnant populations) (see Table 8.1 for FDA categories). A review of 250 medications showed that fewer than 60 were in FDA categories A or B (www.perinatology.com), meaning they had no evidence of risk in humans during pregnancy. This lack of data leaves both patients and providers in a quandary about how to evaluate the risk/benefit ratio for a candidate medication. What should patients and providers do if the pregnant patient must use this medication to protect the quality of her life?

Most estimates of risk for medications used during pregnancy weigh heavily on the health of the fetus and result from case reports or retrospective case-control epidemiological studies. These types of reports are of limited utility due to the potential for reporting bias: negative outcomes are more likely to be reported than uneventful outcomes (American Academy of Pediatrics, 2000). Case reports and retrospective studies are generally limited in the strength of their conclusions due to the lack of control over confounding variables such as maternal age, nutrition, and comorbid physical and psychiatric status; use of nicotine, alcohol, or illicit drugs; misuse of prescribed drugs; environmental toxins; pregnancy history; genetic history; gestational age at time of drug exposure and quantity and frequency of drug exposure during each trimester;

Table 8-1. FDA RATINGS OF MEDICATIONS FOR USE IN PREGNANT PATIENTS

CATEGORY	DEFINITION
A	No risk shown in controlled trials. Adequate, well-controlled studies in pregnant women have failed to demonstrate risk to the fetus.
B	No demonstration of risk in humans. Either animal findings show risk, but human findings do not, or if no adequate human studies have been done, animal findings are negative.
C	Risk is possible. Human studies are lacking, and animal studies are either positive for fetal risk or lacking as well. However, potential benefits may justify the potential risk.
D	Positive evidence of risk. Data show risk to the fetus. Nevertheless, potential benefits may outweigh the potential risk.
X	Contraindicated in pregnancy. Studies in animals or humans, or investigational or post-marketing reports have shown fetal risk that clearly outweighs any possible benefit to the patient.

adherence to the medication regimen; total medication dose; interaction of the medication with other substances; and the effects of the psychiatric illness or other illnesses present. It is highly likely that our collective knowledge regarding the risks of exposure to psychoactive drugs during pregnancy will remain limited due to the ethical standards required by randomized controlled trials.

Because of the potential for physical and behavioral teratogenesis, varying degrees of concern exist when any drug is prescribed during pregnancy (Vorhees et al., 1982). Common advice given to medical providers and pregnant patients is that medications should be avoided as much as possible during pregnancy to prevent embryonic and fetal drug exposure. Such advice is based on the risk of medications producing physical changes in bodily structures (e.g., malformation of limbs, organs, etc.), changes in brain chemistry that produce functional alterations in behavior, as well as other adverse events in the fetus or newborn. However, as with psychiatric disorders, the dangers of failure to treat and the benefits of appropriate psychoactive substance use treatment have been clearly established (e.g., Altshuler et al., 1996).

Medication treatment is indicated if behavioral treatments are either inadequate or inappropriate for the patient's disorder. Wisner et al. (2000) has outlined a decision model that lists the components of a comprehensive discussion for treatment of depression during pregnancy. This model can help the provider and the patient to make an informed decision on treatment options in pregnancy. The provider should discuss with the patient (1) the risk for teratogenic or negative effects for the fetus during the first trimester and (2) whether starting the medication later in the pregnancy would improve the risk/benefit profile.

Once the decision to offer medication is made, important factors in medication selection are listed in Table 8.2.

The body of evidence in the literature to date suggests that many psychotropic drugs are relatively safe to take during pregnancy, and women and their health care providers should not be unduly concerned if a woman requires treatment. Optimal control of the psychiatric disorder should be maintained during pregnancy, the postpartum period, and thereafter. All pregnancies in which an expectant mother has a serious psychiatric disorder should be considered high risk and the mother and fetus must be carefully monitored (Einarson, 2009).

MEDICATION TREATMENT FOR DEPRESSION

Compared to behavioral treatments, a somewhat larger body of research exists on the use of medications to treat nonpregnant women with depression who also have substance use disorders. The results of a meta-analysis on this topic suggested that when medication effectively treats depression, it also reduces substance use (Nunes & Levin, 2004). A more recent study has also concluded that adequate treatment for depression reduces substance use disorders and that the

Table 8-2. FACTORS TO CONSIDER IN ASSESSING THE RISK/BENEFIT RATIO

RISKS
- **Risks to Consider for Embryo, Fetus, and Neonate**
    - **If medication is provided, will the candidate medication produce:**
    Structural malformations
    Intrauterine fetal death
    Altered fetal growth
    Acute neonatal effects (direct drug toxicity or effects of withdrawal from the medication) Neurobehavioral teratogenicity (long-term central nervous system defects that compromise lifelong learning)
    - **If medication is not provided**
    Adverse impact of illness on fetus/neonate
- **Risks to Consider for Mother**
    - **If medication is provided**
    Side effect(s) of the candidate medication for the mother
    Will any of these side effects trigger relapse or otherwise compromise drug abstinence?
    Will the effects of the drug itself trigger relapse?
    Interaction of the candidate medication with any medication the patient may already be taking for drug abstinence (e.g., methadone for opioid dependence)
    Efficacy of the candidate medication
    - **If medication is not provided**
    Potentially life-threatening signs and symptoms
    Less healthy mother less able to comply with prenatal care and/or care of infant
    Worse substance use disorder treatment outcomes
    Impact of maternal illness on fetus/neonate

BENEFITS
▶ **Mother**
  • **Medication treatment**
    Control of potentially life-threatening signs and symptoms
    Healthier mother better able to comply with prenatal/parenting recommendations
    Better substance use disorder treatment outcomes
  • **No medication treatment**
    Avoidance of exposure to medication; thus, reduced chance of side effects
▶ **Fetus/neonate**
  • **Medication treatment**
    Less stress to fetus and optimal mother–child interaction
  • **No medication treatment**
    Elimination of risk of teratogenic and direct toxic effects on fetus/neonate

treatment of substance use disorders has been found to reduce depression (e.g., Davis et al., 2008). The selective serotonin reuptake inhibitors (SSRIs) were found to be first-line medications for nonpregnant patients based on their tolerability and low toxicity relative to tricyclic antidepressants (TCAs). A recent review suggested that the efficacy of integrated treatments remains uncertain given the limited data in this area and the methodological challenges that limit the confidence in reaching strong conclusions from the existing data (Tiet & Mausbach, 2007). Information is clearly lacking regarding the impact that the interaction between medications to treat depression and medications to treat substance use disorders may have on patient outcomes in the treatment of either disorder.

The following paragraphs provide some examples of medications used to treat depression during pregnancy.

For pregnant women, TCAs such as amitriptyline (Elavil), butriptyline (Evadyne), clomipramine (Anafranil), doxepin (Adapin, Sinequan), imipramine (Tofranil), lofepramine (Lomont, Gamanil), and trimipramine (Surmontil) are not the medications of first choice for treating depression. They have been associated with congenital heart malformations, transient neonatal adverse effects (e.g., Källén & Otterblad Olausson, 2006), and uncomfortable maternal side effects. With newer medication options to treat depression, such as SSRIs, fewer prescriptions for TCAs have been written for pregnant women.

TCAs can also be problematic in conjunction with the use of methadone during pregnancy. For example, TCAs, methadone, and pregnancy each cause constipation, making the need for fiber and stool softeners important. Dry mouth is also a side effect of TCAs, so patients maintained on TCAs need to regularly brush their teeth and drink water and avoid sugar and sodas to maintain dental health. One TCA, desipramine (Norpramin), results in increased medication blood levels when methadone is initiated (Maany et al., 1989) because methadone reduces the metabolism of desipramine (Kosten et al., 1992).

Prenatal exposure to SSRIs (e.g., fluoxetine, sertraline, paroxetine, fluvoxamine) and other newer antidepressants (bupropion, mirtazapine, venlafaxine, nefazadone) has received considerable scientific attention. There is a rapidly growing body of literature on their use, with contradictory conclusions. The most recent meta-analysis concluded that SSRIs increase the risk of spontaneous abortion but not the risk of malformations (heart or others; Rahimi et al., 2006). Another study showed that smoking 10 or more cigarettes/day and first-trimester fluoxetine exposure were the only significant variables for cardiovascular anomalies (Diav-Citrin et al., 2008). It is possible that the birth anomalies were related to the actual illness of depression, smoking, or medication exposure, or any combination. Therefore, patients should be counseled about reducing cigarette smoking, and depression must be treated.

Fluoxetine (Prozac) has been repeatedly shown to be associated with neonatal toxicity and possibly a withdrawal syndrome comprising jitteriness, jaundice, and hypoglycemia (Mhanna et al., 1997). There is also evidence of persistent pulmonary hypertension (Chambers et al., 1996) associated with the regular use of fluoxetine. There do not appear to be long-term developmental effects of prenatal exposure to fluoxetine (Nulman et al., 1997, 2002). While limiting fetal exposure to drugs and medications is important, minimizing fetal exposure to the depressive illness is also critical. The individual patient and provider must weigh the risk/benefit ratio of medication treatment during pregnancy.

Paroxetine (Paxil, Aropax, Seroxat) should be avoided in women who are planning to become pregnant or women in their first trimester due to the very small (1%) but important potential for congenital effects (see the American Congress of Obstetricians and Gynecologists website for details). There is also the risk of maternal or neonatal withdrawal if medication is abruptly discontinued (Misri & Kendrick, 2007). After delivery, jitteriness, irritability, vomiting, seizures, respiratory distress, hypotonia, and other abnormalities of neonatal adaptation may occur among infants whose mothers are treated with paroxetine late in pregnancy (Davis et al., 2007; Moses-Kolko et al., 2005; Way, 2007). Neonatal drug withdrawal or paroxetine toxicity may be responsible for these neonatal issues. Altered pain response has been reported in infants whose mothers were maintained on paroxetine during pregnancy (Oberlander et al., 2002).

Monoamine oxidase inhibitors (MAOIs) should be avoided in patients using cocaine and/or alcohol and/or using or treated with opioids. Severe to fatal interactions can occur due to an interaction between MAOIs and these latter substances. Furthermore, MAOIs should be avoided in pregnancy due to an association with fetal growth restriction (Briggs et al., 2008).

MEDICATION TREATMENT FOR ANXIETY

Benzodiazepines should be avoided in the treatment of anxiety in patients also being treated for substance use disorders due to the high risk of abuse. The importance of avoiding these medications in pregnant patients with substance use disorders is compounded by the small but significant risk of birth defects associated with benzodiazepine use (Howland, 2009).

TEMPORAL PARADIGMS FOR TREATMENT

There are three paradigms for treating pregnant women with substance use and comorbid psychiatric disorders: parallel, sequential, and integrated (Drake et al., 2001). The integrated model of care is the preferred model of care and the standard of care. In the integrated model, patients have higher rates of adherence to treatment and improved clinical outcomes compared to patients receiving parallel or sequential treatment (Mueser et al., 2003).

PRACTICAL STRATEGIES FOR FACILITATING TREATMENT ENTRY AND ADHERENCE AND COORDINATING TREATMENT SERVICES

A number of strategies exist to increase the likelihood that patients will enter treatment, engage in it, and remain in it (Daley & Marlatt, 2006; Rollnick, Miller, & Butler, 2007). Specific strategies can be found in Table 8.3 (see Chapter 6 for more information).

As discussed in Chapter 6, the treatment clinic should have patients sign a form giving the program permission to require independent evaluation if there is concern about the patient's care or if there is concern that not all information

Table 8-3. STRATEGIES FOR HELPING PATIENTS ACCEPT
THE REFERRAL TO ADDITIONAL CARE

- Using Motivational Interviewing techniques, assess patient's motivation to start treatment for comorbid psychiatric disorder and then address patient's ambivalence about treatment.
- Frame referral for treatment in positive manner and explain how treating the comorbid disorder may make drug treatment more successful.
- Use reminder phone calls or letters before initial visit.
- Give date and time of appointment to the patient in writing.
- Assess the barriers to attending the appointment and then strategize with the patient about how to overcome each barrier.
- Provide as much information as possible using concrete items like pictures, brochures, flyers, etc. about what the program or service is, what it is like to be there, and what to expect from the treatment. Role-play with the patient about how she will ask questions about the program or service, or role-play other aspects that are concerning to the patient.
- Use any and all support resources (e.g., family members, drug-free friends, NA sponsor) the patient may have available to her to reinforce the need for and entry into treatment.
- Negotiate a behavioral contract with the patient stating the number of visits she will make to the new service before deciding on its usefulness.
- As soon as possible after the day of the scheduled appointment, follow up with the patient to ensure the appointment was kept. If the appointment was missed, find out why and discuss plans for a new appointment. If the appointment was kept, provide verbal praise and discuss the next appointment and the patient's experience with the service in terms of the likelihood that she will continue attending.
- Know the date and time of each appointment. Monitor whether the patient attends and provide feedback (positive or corrective) accordingly.

related to the patient's situation and care is being shared. At treatment intake and as soon as outside treatment is known, the substance use treatment clinic staff should have permission to exchange information with the outside providers to discuss the patient's case.

SUMMARY

In the pregnant patient with a substance use disorder, treatment of any comorbid psychiatric disorders must be conducted in a manner integrated with the treatment for substance use disorder. When considering psychotropic medications for use in this population, providers must carefully review the risks and benefits of the candidate treatment.

REFERENCES

Altshuler, L. L., Cohen, L., Szuba, M. P., Burt, V. K., Gitlin, M., & Mintz, J. (1996). Pharmacologic management of psychiatric illness during pregnancy: dilemmas and guidelines. *American Journal of Psychiatry,153*(5), 592–606.

American Academy of Pediatrics, Committee on Drugs. (2000). Use of psychoactive medication during pregnancy and possible effects on the fetus and newborn. *Pediatrics,105*(4 Pt 1), 880–887.

American Psychiatric Association. (1995). *Diagnostic and statistical manual of mental disorders* (4th ed.). Washington, D.C.: American Psychiatric Association.

Battle, C. L., Zlotnick, C., Miller, I. W., Pearlstein, T., & Howard, M. (2006). Clinical characteristics of perinatal psychiatric patients: a chart review study. *Journal of Nervous and Mental Disease, 194,* 369–377.

Bennett, H. A., Einarson, A., Taddio, A., Koren, G., & Einarson, T. R. (2004). Depression during pregnancy: Overview of clinical factors. *Clinical Drug Investigation, 24*(3), 157–179.

Benningfield, M. M., Dietrich, M. S., Jones, H. E., Kaltenbach, K., Heil, S. H., Stine, S. M., Coyle, M. G., Arria, A. M., O'Grady, K. E., Fischer, G., & Martin, P. R. (2012). Opioid dependence during pregnancy: relationships of depression and anxiety symptoms to treatment outcomes. *Addiction, 107(Suppl. 1),* 74–82.

Briggs, G. G., Freeman, R. K., & Yaffe, S. J. (2008). *Drugs in pregnancy and lactation* (8th ed.). Philadelphia, PA: Lippincott William & Wilkins.

Burns, K., Melamed, J., Burns, W., Chasnoff, I., & Hatcher, R. (1985). Chemical dependence and clinical depression in pregnancy. *Journal of Clinical Psychology, 41,* 851–854.

Chambers, C. D., Johnson, K. A., Dick, L. M., Felix, R. J., & Jones, K. L. (1996). Birth outcomes in pregnant women taking fluoxetine. *New England Journal of Medicine, 335*(14), 1010–1050.

Cohen, L. S., Nonacs, R. M., Bailey, J. W., Viguera, A. C., Reminick, A. M., Altshuler, L. L., Stowe, Z. N., & Faraone, S. V. (2004). Relapse of depression during pregnancy following antidepressant discontinuation: a preliminary prospective study. *Archives of Women's Mental Health, 7*(4), 217–221.

Daley, D. C., & Marlatt, A. G. (2006). *Overcoming your alcohol or drug problem: Effective recovery strategies.* New York: Oxford University Press.

Davis, L., Uezato, A., Newell, J. M., & Frazier, E. (2008). Major depression and comorbid substance use disorders. *Current Opinion in Psychiatry, 21*(1), 14–18.

Davis, L. L., Frazier, E. C., Gaynes, B. N., Trivedi, M. H., Wisniewski, S. R., Fava, M., Barkin, J., Kashner, T. M., Shelton, R. C., Alpert, J. E., & Rush, A. J. (2007). Are depressed outpatients with and without a family history of substance use disorder different? A baseline analysis of the STAR*D cohort. *Journal of Clinical Psychiatry, 68*(12), 1931–1938.

Diav-Citrin, O., Shechtman, S., Weinbaum, D., Wajnberg, R., Avgil, M., Di Gianantonio, E., Clementi, M., Weber-Schoendorfer, C., Schaefer, C., & Ornoy, A. (2008). Paroxetine and fluoxetine in pregnancy: a prospective, multicentre, controlled, observational study. *British Journal of Clinical Pharmacology, 66*(5), 695–705.

Diego, M. A., Field, T., Hernandez-Reif, M., Cullen, C., Schanberg, S., & Kuhn, C. (2004). Prepartum, postpartum, and chronic depression effects on newborns. *Psychiatry, 67,* 63–80.

Diego, M. A., Field, T., Hernandez-Reif, M., Schanberg, S., Kuhn, C., & Gonzalez-Quintero, V. H. (2009). Prenatal depression restricts fetal growth. *Early Human Development, 85* (1), 65–70.

Drake, R. E., Essock, S. M., Shaner, A., Carey, K. B., Minkoff, K., Kola, L., Lynde, D., Osher, F. C., Clark, R. E., & Rickards, L. (2001). Implementing dual diagnosis services for clients with severe mental illness. *Psychiatric Services, 52*(4), 469–476.

Einarson, A. (2009). Introduction: reproductive mental health—Motherisk update 2008. *Canadian Journal of Clinical Pharmacology, 16*(1), e1–e5.

Field, T., Diego, M., & Hernandez-Reif, M. (2008). Prenatal dysthymia versus major depression effects on the neonate. *Infant Behavior and Development, 31*(2) 190–193.

Field, T., Diego, M., Hernandez-Reif, M., & Fernandez, M. (2007). Depressed mothers' newborns show less discrimination of other newborns' cry sounds. *Infant Behavior and Development, 30*(3), 431–435.

Field, T., Diego, M., Hernandez-Reif, M., Figueiredo, B., Schanberg, S., Kuhn, C., Deeds, O., Contogeorgos, J., & Ascencio, A. (2008). Chronic prenatal depression and neonatal outcome. *International Journal of Neuroscience, 118*(1), 95–103.

Finnegan, L. P. (1981). The effects of narcotics and alcohol on pregnancy and the newborn. *Annals of the New York Academy of Sciences, 362,* 136–157.

First, M. B., Gibbon, M., Spitzer, R. L., Williams, J. B. W., & Benjamin, L.S. (1997). *Structured Clinical Interview for DSM-IV Axis II Personality Disorders (SCID-II).* Washington, DC: American Psychiatric Press.

Fitzsimons, H. E., Tuten, M., Vaidya, V., & Jones, H. E. (2007). Mood disorders affect drug treatment success of drug-dependent pregnant women. *Journal of Substance Abuse Treatment, 32*(1), 19–25.

Gavin, N. I., Gaynes, B. N., Lohr, K. N., Meltzer-Brody, S., Gartlehner, G., & Swinson, T. (2005). Perinatal depression: a systematic review of prevalence and incidence. *Obstetrics & Gynecology, 106*(5 Pt 1), 1071–1083.

Grote, N. K., Bridge, J. A., Gavin, A. R., Melville, J. L., Iyengar, S., & Katon, W. J. (2010). A meta-analysis of depression during pregnancy and the risk of preterm birth, low birth weight, and intrauterine growth restriction. *Archives of General Psychiatry, 67*(10), 1012–1024.

Haller, D. L., Knisely, J. S., Dawson, K. S., & Schnoll, S. H. (1993). Perinatal substance abusers: Psychological and social characteristics. *Journal of Nervous and Mental Disease, 181*(8), 509–513.

Haller, D. L., Miles, D. R., & Dawson, K. S. (2002). Psychopathology influences treatment retention among drug-dependent women. *Journal of Substance Abuse Treatment, 23*(4), 431–436.

Holbrook, A., & Kaltenbach, K. (2012). Co-occurring psychiatric symptoms in opioid-dependent women: the prevalence of antenatal and postnatal depression. *American Journal of Drug and Alcohol Abuse, 38(6), 575–579.*

Hollon, S. D., DeRubeis, R. J., Evans Wiemer, M. J., Garvey, M. J., Grove, W. M., & Tuason, V. B. (1992). Cognitive therapy and pharmacotherapy for depression: Singly and in combination. *Archives of General Psychiatry, 49*(10), 774–781.

Howland, R. H. (2009). Prescribing psychotropic medications during pregnancy and lactation: Principles and guidelines. *Journal of Psychosocial Nursing and Mental Health Services, 47*(5), 19–23.

Källén, B., & Otterblad Olausson, P. (2006). Antidepressant drugs during pregnancy and infant congenital heart defect. *Reproductive Toxicology, 21*(3), 221–222.

Kessler, R. C., Davis, C. G., & Kendler, K. S. (1997). Childhood adversity and adult psychiatric disorder in the US National Comorbidity Survey. *Psychological Medicine, 25*(5), 1101–1119.

King, V. L., & Brooner, R. K. (1999). Assessment and treatment of comorbid psychiatric disorders. In E. Strain & M. Stitzer (Eds.), *Methadone treatment for opioid dependence.* Baltimore: Johns Hopkins University Press.

Kissin, W. B., Svikis, D. S., Morgan, G. D., & Haug, N. A. (2001). Characterizing pregnant drug-dependent women in treatment and their children. *Journal of Substance Abuse Treatment, 21*(1), 27–34.

Kosten, T. R., Morgan, C. M., Falcione, J., & Schottenfeld, R. S. (1992). Pharmacotherapy for cocaine-abusing methadone-maintained patients using amantadine or desipramine. *Archives of General Psychiatry, 49*(11), 894–898.

Littleton, H. L., Breitkopf, C. R., & Berenson, A. B. (2007). Correlates of anxiety symptoms during pregnancy and association with perinatal outcomes: A meta-analysis. *American Journal of Obstetrics and Gynecology, 196*(5), 424–432.

Maany, I., Dhopesh, V., Arndt, I. O., Burke, W., Woody, G., & O'Brien, C. P. (1989). Increase in desipramine serum levels associated with methadone treatment. *American Journal of Psychiatry, 146*(12), 1611–1613.

Martin, P. R., Arria, A. M., Fischer, G., Kaltenbach, K., Heil, S. H., Stine, S. M., Coyle, M. G., Selby, P., & Jones, H. E. (2009). Psychopharmacologic management of opioid-dependent women during pregnancy. *American Journal on Addictions, 18*(2), 148–156.

Mhanna, M. J., Bennet, J. B. II, & Izatt, S. D. (1997). Potential fluoxetine chloride (Prozac) toxicity in a newborn. *Journal of the American Academy of Pediatrics, 100,* 158–159.

Misri, S., & Kendrick, K. (2007). Treatment of perinatal mood and anxiety disorders: A review. *Canadian Journal of Psychiatry, 52*(8), 489–498.

Moses-Kolko, E. L., Bogen, D., Perel, J., Bregar, A., Uhl, K., Levin, B., & Wisner, K. L. (2005). Neonatal signs after late in utero exposure to serotonin reuptake inhibitors: Literature review and implications for clinical applications. *Journal of the American Medical Association, 293*(19), 2372–2383.

Moylan, P. L., Jones, H. E., Haug, N. A., Kissin, W. B., & Svikis, D. S. (2001). Clinical and psychosocial characteristics of substance-dependent pregnant women with and without PTSD. *Addictive Behaviors, 26*(3), 469–474.

Mueser, K. T., Torrey, W. C., Lynde, D., Singer, P., & Drake, R. E. (2003). Implementing evidence-based practices for people with severe mental illness. *Behavioral Modification, 27*(3), 387–411.

Nemeroff, C. B., Bremner, J. D., Foa, E. B., Mayberg, H. S., North, C. S., & Stein, M. B. (2006). Posttraumatic stress disorder: A state-of-the-science review. *Journal of Psychiatric Research, 40*(1), 1–21.

Newport, D. J., Ji, S., Long, Q., Knight, B. T., Zach, E. B., Smith, E. N., Morris, N. J., & Stowe, Z. N. (2012). Maternal depression and anxiety differentially impact fetal exposures during pregnancy. *Journal of Clinical Psychiatry, 73*(2), 247–251.

Nulman, I., Rovet, J., Stewart, D. E., Wolpin, J., Gardner, H. A., Theis, J. G., Kulin, N., & Koren, G. (1997). Neurodevelopment of children exposed in utero to antidepressant drugs. *New England Journal of Medicine, 336*(4), 258–262.

Nulman, I., Rovet, J., Stewart, D. E., Wolpin, J., Pace-Asciak, P., Shuhaiber, S., & Koren, G. (2002). Child development following exposure to tricyclic antidepressants or fluoxetine throughout fetal life: A prospective, controlled study. *American Journal of Psychiatry, 159*(11), 1889–1895.

Nunes, E. V., & Levin, F. R. (2004). Treatment of depression in patients with alcohol or other drug dependence: A meta-analysis. *Journal of the American Medical Association, 291*(15), 1887–1896.

Oberlander, T. F., Eckstein Grunau, R., Fitzgerald, C., Ellwood, A. L., Misri, S., Rurak, D., & Riggs, K. W. (2002). Prolonged prenatal psychotropic medication exposure alters neonatal acute pain response. *Pediatric Research, 51*(4), 443–453.

Perkonigg, A., Kessler, R. C., Storz, S., & Wittchen, H. U. (2000). Traumatic events and post-traumatic stress disorder in the community: Prevalence, risk factors and comorbidity. *Acta Psychiatrica Scandinavica, 101*(1), 46–59.

Rahimi, R., Nikfar, S., & Abdollahi, M. (2006). Pregnancy outcomes following exposure to serotonin reuptake inhibitors: A meta-analysis of clinical trials. *Reproductive Toxicology, 22*(4), 571–575.

Rollnick, S., Miller, W. R., & Butler, C. C. (2007). *Motivational interviewing in health care: Helping patients change behavior.* New York: The Guilford Press.

Rosen, D., Seng, J. S., Tolman, R. M., & Mallinger, G. (2007). Intimate partner violence, depression, and posttraumatic stress disorder as additional predictors of low birth weight infants among low-income mothers. *Journal of Interpersonal Violence, 22*(10), 1305–1314.

Schetter, C., & Tanner, L. (2012). Anxiety, depression and stress in pregnancy: implications for mothers, children, research, and practice. *Current Opinion Psychiatry, 25*(2), 141–148.

Seng, J. S., Low, L. K., Sperlich, M., Ronis, D. L., & Liberzon, I. (2011). Post-traumatic stress disorder, child abuse history, birthweight and gestational age: a prospective cohort study. *British Journal of Obstetrics & Gynaecology, 118*(11), 1329–1339.

Seng, J. S., Oakley, D. J., Sampselle, C. M., Killion, C., Graham-Bermann, S., & Liberzon I. (2001). Posttraumatic stress disorder and pregnancy complications. *Obstetrics and Gynecology, 97*(1), 17–22.

Tiet, Q. Q., & Mausbach, B. (2007). Treatments for patients with dual diagnosis: A review. *Alcoholism: Clinical and Experimental Research, 31*(4), 513–536.

Tuten, M., Heil, S., O'Grady, K. E., Fitzsimons, H., Chisolm, M., & Jones, H. E. (2009). Methadone-maintained pregnant patients and current mood disorder: Delivery and neonatal outcomes. *American Journal of Drug and Alcohol Abuse, 35*(5), 358–363.

Vesga-López, O., Blanco, C., Keyes, K., Olfson, M., Grant, B. F., & Hasin, D. S. (2008). Psychiatric disorders in pregnant and postpartum women in the United States. *Archives of General Psychiatry, 65*(7), 805–815.

Vorhees, C. V., Klein, K. L., & Scott, W. J. (1982). Aspirin-induced psychoteratogenesis in rats as a function of embryonic age. *Teratogenesis, Carcinogenesis, and Mutagenesis, 2*(1), 77–84.

Way, C. M. (2007). Safety of newer antidepressants in pregnancy. *Pharmacotherapy, 24*(4), 546–552.

Weiss, R. D. (2004). Treating patients with bipolar disorder and substance dependence: Lessons learned. *Journal of Substance Abuse Treatment, 27*(4), 307–312.

Wisner, K. L., Zarin, D. A., Holmboe, E. S., Appelbaum, P. S., Gelenberg, A. J., Leonard, H. L., & Frank, E. (2000). Risk-benefit decision making for treatment of depression during pregnancy. *American Journal of Psychiatry, 157*(12), 1933–1940.

Zuckerman, B., Bauchner, H., Parker, S., & Cabral, H. (1990). Maternal depressive symptoms during pregnancy, and newborn irritability. *Journal of Developmental & Behavioral Pediatrics, 11*(4), 190–194.

9

Understanding the Obstetrical Aspects of Care of the Pregnant Woman with Substance Use Disorders

OVERVIEW

I n this chapter we review the medical and obstetrical complications characteristic of pregnant women with substance use disorders and issues regarding the provision of prenatal care. We discuss the clinical management of this population, as well as the need to provide extensive prenatal and obstetrical education and nutritional counseling. We give examples of recommended laboratory tests, assessments, referral services, and educational information. We highlight the importance of pain management during and after delivery. Finally, a summary of the chapter is presented to emphasize its key points.

INTRODUCTION

Pregnant women with substance use disorders often have an array of medical and obstetrical complications due to their life circumstances and their lack of health care. Most often they enter treatment after many years of chronic substance use; their lives may include homelessness or transient housing that involves living with friends or relatives; poverty; exchanging sex for food/shelter or drugs; commercial sex work; and poor nutrition. Related to their substance use disorder, they have not sought preventive health care and have neglected their acute health care needs. Any experiences with health care providers that they have had may have ranged from unpleasant to appalling to frightening, as women with substance use disorders in general—and pregnant women with substance use disorders in particular—are frequently viewed with disrespect and even contempt. Previous experiences and/or her own behavior that may be socially unacceptable can generate a cycle of distrust and lack of engagement on the part of the patient and unsupportive and judgmental behavior on the part of the health care provider. A pregnant woman with a substance use disorder who is treated rudely by a clerk checking her in to prenatal care may become confrontational, a behavior that reinforces staff expectations that she is a difficult and problematic patient before she even enters the examining room.

MEDICAL COMPLICATIONS

Although there are medical complications associated with specific drugs, it is rare that a pregnant woman's substance use disorder will include only one drug. For example, alcohol is often combined with nicotine; cocaine is often used with nicotine, alcohol, marijuana, and/or opioids; opioids are used with nicotine, alcohol, cocaine, and/or benzodiazepines. As a result, there are both multiple medical risks and cumulative medical risks due to concomitant substance use.

Smoking tobacco increases a woman's risk for heart disease and lung and esophageal cancer. Women who have the hepatitis B virus and smoke are at increased risk for cervical cancer (CDC, 1989). Cocaine increases the risk for cardiac arrest, and crack cocaine is associated with respiratory and pulmonary disease, as is marijuana. Women who abuse alcohol have an increased risk for circulatory and cardiovascular disorders and cirrhosis of the liver. There is also some concern that they may be at increased risk for breast cancer (Gordis, 1990). Intravenous substance use (most often heroin) historically has been associated with increased incidence of infections, including bacterial endocarditis (Cherubin et al., 1968), cellulitis (Naeye et al., 1973), and tetanus (Cherubin, 1971). However, these data predate the use of opioid agonist treatment (e.g., methadone and buprenorphine) for opioid dependence. A recent study (Holbrook et al., 2012) of pregnant women receiving medication-assisted treatment for opioid dependence found infectious medical complications such as cellulitis and syphilis to be very infrequent, and there was no incidence of bacterial endocarditis or tetanus. Both opioid and cocaine abuse are associated with sexually transmitted diseases, cervical cancer, hepatitis B and C, and HIV. As discussed in Chapter 5, pregnant women entering treatment must undergo a complete medical evaluation so that health issues can be fully addressed. Improving the overall health of the woman is vital not only for a healthy pregnancy but for successful treatment and recovery outcomes.

OBSTETRICAL COMPLICATIONS

Obstetrical complications that occur in pregnant women with substance use disorders are similar to those observed in pregnant women who do not receive prenatal care, such as spontaneous abortion, stillbirth, placental insufficiency, intrauterine growth retardation, premature labor/delivery, premature rupture of membranes, anemia, preeclampsia, and abruptio placentae (Curet & Hsi, 2002; Finnegan, 1979). Therefore, pregnant women with substance use disorders must receive appropriate screening and assessment, as described in Chapters 4 and 5. They must be engaged in treatment services as early in gestation as possible, and treatment programs must provide coordinated services that include both prenatal care and substance use treatment. When women receive prenatal care in conjunction with substance use treatment, obstetrical complications have been found to be infrequent (Holbrook et al., 2012).

Coordinated services can be provided in different settings: prenatal and obstetrical care can be integrated within a comprehensive substance use treatment program (Finnegan, Hagan, & Kaltenbach, 1991), or substance use treatment can be part of a comprehensive perinatal care program for women in treatment for substance disorders (Curet et al., 2002). Chapter 11 delineates the components of comprehensive care recommended for this special population.

OBSTETRICAL CARE

Whether the setting for obstetrical care is a comprehensive substance use treatment program, a prenatal care program that includes substance use treatment, or a coordination of services between a substance use treatment program and an obstetrical clinic, services must be provided in a supportive, nonjudgmental, nonthreatening environment. Staff must treat the pregnant woman who has a substance use disorder with the same respect and concern for her well-being that is given to all other pregnant women. Directives should always be given with basic explanations as to why, what, when, and where. All staff, be it clerical support, nurses, or physicians, should provide gentle encouragement, supportive reminders, and positive reinforcement for keeping appointments and arriving for them on time, exhibiting appropriate behavior, and complying with prenatal care.

While provision of prenatal services is recommended for all programs providing treatment to pregnant women, it is required for pregnant women receiving medication-assisted treatment (i.e., methadone) from a licensed opioid treatment program. Under federal methadone regulations, 42CFR8.12, pregnant women must be given priority for admittance to an opioid treatment program, and the program must, at a minimum, coordinate prenatal care with a medical provider if it does not have the capacity to provide obstetrical services. This coordination can be accomplished by establishing communication between the treatment program and the woman's obstetrician, entering a Memorandum of Understanding with a local obstetrical practice/clinic, coordinating services with local public health clinics, etc. With a Consent to Release Information to both entities, two-way communication can allow the obstetrician to know how engaged the woman is in her substance use treatment, her current methadone dose, prescribed psychiatric medications, and the results of random urine drug screenings; conversely, the medical director of the treatment program will have information regarding compliance with prenatal care, any medical issues that may have an bearing on methadone and/or other medication management, treatment engagement and retention, and successful recovery. Federal regulation 42CFR8.12 applies only to opioid treatment programs; it does not apply to buprenorphine-certified physicians prescribing buprenorphine within an office-based practice. However, all physicians involved in the care of an opioid-dependent pregnant woman whose substance use disorder is being treated with methadone or buprenorphine must be aware of all prescribed medications and illicit drugs she is consuming and must ensure that she receives appropriate prenatal care.

A key component in facilitating and coordinating obstetrical services within a treatment program is having a designated staff member who serves as a liaison between patients, obstetrical staff, program medical staff, and program clinical staff. Nurses or case managers may be the most appropriate staff for this role.

CLINICAL MANAGEMENT

One of the most difficult issues in coordinating obstetrical services is overcoming the stigma, lack of knowledge, and misconceptions related to pregnant women with substance use disorders. Establishing collaborative relationships among patients and staff is often impeded by medical staff's lack of knowledge about the behavioral manifestations of the disease of addiction. Stigma and prejudice can foster an environment of alienation, confrontational interactions, and maladaptive responses to typical behaviors exhibited by patients. Advocacy and education by the staff liaison to decrease stigma and promote care delivered with dignity and respect is the first step to creating a meaningful collaboration between substance use treatment and obstetrical services and the patient.

Information to be presented by the liaison person may include treatment program policies, stages of recovery and how unrealistic staff expectations may affect relationships and interactions, typical psychiatric and social issues of the population, and positive engagement strategies. Effective interventions include role-playing common negative interaction scenarios; educating staff and patients about anger management techniques; providing consistent reinforcement of open communication channels between the treatment program, obstetrical clinic, hospital labor and delivery department, and maternal and nursery nursing staff; establishing open forum problem solving; and developing a mutually supportive relationship with hospital social workers.

Some additional training sessions and interventions are necessary when providing medication-assisted treatment to opioid-dependent pregnant women. All staff, physicians, nurses, and hospital social workers must understand the benefits and risks of medication-assisted treatment during pregnancy, medication dosing, and appropriate pain management for delivery and postoperative care. It is also important to collaborate with nursery staff and mutually develop appropriate maternal behavioral expectations that will promote positive experiences for both mother and nursery staff, especially when infants require treatment for neonatal abstinence syndrome (see Chapter 10).

Table 9.1 gives examples of recommended laboratory tests, Table 9.2 lists recommended assessments, and Table 9.3 lists possible referral services for pregnant patients with substance use disorders.

PRENATAL EDUCATION

In addition to medical care, patients will need specific educational information about several issues.

It is helpful to discuss with the patient the scope of prenatal care in terms of what to expect at each visit and the reasons for certain procedures and tests. The discussion should also include the specific risks of substance use, and particularly drug interactions (e.g., methadone and benzodiazepines). Prenatal health education should be provided through classes conducted by nursing staff, videos, and/or printed booklets. Any printed materials must be written at the appropriate reading level for patients.

Opioid-dependent pregnant patients maintained on methadone or buprenorphine should be informed of the need to ingest increased fiber a stool softener to counteract the constipation associated with taking methadone or buprenorphine.

Opioid-dependent pregnant patients should have a thorough understanding of the risks and benefits of medication-assisted treatment in pregnancy. The adequacy of the methadone or buprenorphine dose should be discussed so that the patient understands the difference between symptoms of withdrawal and normal discomforts of pregnancy; how a therapeutic dose varies

Table 9-1. RECOMMENDED LABORATORY TESTS

- Complete blood count with differential and platelets
- Repeat complete blood count and serology at 24 to 28 weeks
- SMA-12 blood test
- Rapid plasma reagin (RPR) serology and testing for gonorrhea and chlamydia
- Blood type: RH and indirect Coombs
- Hepatic panel
- Rubella titer
- Varicella
- PPD tuberculosis skin test
- HIV with counseling by experienced HIV counselor
- Urinalysis (routine and microscopic)
- Urine culture and sensitivity
- Panel 8* urine drug screen
- Hepatitis B surface antigen (full panel if positive)
- Hepatitis C antibody; if positive, HCV viral load by polymerase chain reaction (PCR)
- Liver function tests every trimester for HCV-positive patients
- 1 hour 50 mg glucose challenge test at 24 to 28 weeks (also at initial visit if at risk for gestational diabetes)
- Serum triple screen examination at 18 to 22 weeks for detection of fetal anomalies
- Group B streptococcus (GBS) vaginal-rectal culture at 35 to 37 weeks

*Screens for THC (marijuana), cocaine, PCP, opiates, methamphetamines (including Ecstasy), amphetamines, barbiturates, and benzodiazepines. Methadone, buprenorphine, and oxycodone will not be identified under opiates; they must be specifically added to a UDS panel.

Table 9-2. RECOMMENDED ASSESSMENTS

- Full OB physical with Pap test
- Ultrasonographic confirmation of estimated gestational age
- Ultrasonographic examination in third trimester to assess fetal growth
- Nonstress test when intrauterine growth restriction is present
- Assess for presence of trauma
- EKG for baseline and/or follow-up for methadone-maintained patients
- Assess for depression

Table 9-3. POSSIBLE REFERRALS FOR PREGNANT WOMEN WITH
SUBSTANCE USE DISORDERS

▪ HIV-positive patients referred to infectious disease specialist ▪ Hepatitis C-positive patients referred to gastroenterologist/hepatologist ▪ Patients with poor dental health referred to dentist ▪ Patients with history of trauma and/or interpersonal violence referred to appropriate social service and clinical intervention ▪ All eligible patients referred to Women Infants and Children (WIC) nutritional program ▪ All smokers referred to smoking cessation counseling ▪ Patients with co-occurring disorders referred to psychiatric services ▪ Patients with endocarditis or history of endocarditis referred to cardiologist

Referral lists/resources should be provided for treatment services for substance use disorders and treatment for sexually transmitted disease(s) for the patient's partner, when appropriate.

for each individual so that the appropriate dose for her may differ from that of her fellow patients; how her dose may need to be increased as her pregnancy progresses; how to recognize fetal stress if she begins to experience withdrawal; and the risk to both her and her fetus of continued illicit substance use. She should understand that upon delivery her opioid agonist medication dose may need to be tapered down, and she should request a decrease if she feels overly sedated. Chapter 7 provides a thorough discussion of medication-assisted treatment.

OBSTETRICAL EDUCATION

We have found that patients being treated for substance use disorders have a great deal of misinformation about sexuality, pregnancy, labor and delivery, birth control, and breastfeeding. Education about these aspects of care can be provided individually or in group formats. These sessions can also be another arena in which to discuss and role-play sexual empowerment skills (e.g., how to persuade men to wear condoms, how to use female condoms, how to refuse unwanted sexual contact) for negotiating safer sex with partners (Jones et al., 2011). These skills should be taught during HIV risk-reduction education and should be reiterated and reinforced during obstetrical visits.

NUTRITIONAL COUNSELING

Adequate nutrition during pregnancy is built on basic principles and is quite similar to healthy eating at any time in life. Pregnant women should avoid empty calories and junk food. The patient and her fetus require a regular supply of good nutrients. The "right" foods include protein (and the amino acids within) because these nutrients are important building blocks of human cells. Daily protein intake should be about 75 grams. For example, a cheese omelet for breakfast, a hamburger and salad for lunch, and chicken with dinner can provide adequate protein. Grains, legumes, and soy are also good sources of protein. Other vitamins needed for the health of the mother and baby include vitamin C (the body can't store it, so a fresh supply is needed each day to help boost the baby's growth and development and keep the patient's immune system functioning). Orange juice and fruits and vegetables like kiwi, mango, strawberries, melon, bell peppers, tomatoes, and asparagus are good sources of vitamin C. Calcium is critical during pregnancy for the baby's developing bones and for decreasing the risk of osteoporosis later in life. Milk, yogurt, and cheese are good sources of calcium. Remind patients that caffeine and high-fiber foods can slow the absorption of calcium.

Vegetables such as spinach and broccoli, and fruits such as mango and cantaloupe, have more essential vitamins and minerals than most other produce, including vitamin E, riboflavin, folic acid, magnesium, and beta-carotene; these vitamins and minerals are vital to the baby's skin, bones, eyes, and cell growth. Complex carbohydrates (breads, cereals, and pastas) are not only are healthy choices but also combat nausea (from their starchiness) and fight constipation (due to their fiber). Iron is also needed more than ever due to the fetus' rapidly developing blood supply and the mother's expanding blood supply. Iron is found in soy products, beef, dried fruit, and blackstrap molasses, in addition to prenatal supplements.

Fat is vital to the fetus and neonate, in particular omega-3 fatty acids, which fuel proper brain growth and eye development (especially during the third trimester). However, no more than 30% of a day's calories should come from fat. For many women, that means one fast-food burger and fries. Adding salt to meals should be avoided, as most foods already have salt in them. A healthy goal for all adults is approximately 2,400 mg of sodium per day (most Americans consume 4,000 to 8,000 mg daily).

Drinking water is one of the most important behaviors for pregnant women, both for themselves and the baby. As body fluids increase during pregnancy, so does the need for fluid intake. The fetus needs fluid for building body cells, delivering nutrients, and excreting wastes. Extra fluid helps the body get rid of toxins and waste products, keeps toilet habits regular, and reduces the risk of urinary tract infection. Getting plenty of water can also keep the body from retaining too much water. Drinking 2 quarts (64 ounces) a day should be encouraged. If trips to the bathroom are frequent and urine is pale or colorless, then the patient's water intake is sufficient.

PAIN MANAGEMENT

Special attention needs to be paid to managing non-labor pain and labor pain in women with substance use disorders. Pain management during labor and delivery needs to be provided in the safest and most effective ways. Part of pain management includes reassuring the patient that her pain will be addressed. Analgesic needs should be based on the clinical evaluation of the patient. For opioid agonist treated patients, the dose of pain medication should not be reduced due to the prescribed maintenance dose of opioid agonist medication. The dose of agonist medication can continue uninterrupted (Jones et al., 2006, 2009). Full opioid agonists can be used for pain relief in most women with substance use disorders, including those with opioid use disorders. To treat labor pain, epidural analgesia is similarly effective in women with and without opioid use disorders (e.g., Cassidy & Cyna, 2004; Myer et al., 2010). For opioid using or treated women, the use of mixed opioid agonist-antagonists (e.g., nalbuphine or butorphanol) must be avoided as these medications precipitate opioid withdrawal in opioid-using patients.

SUMMARY

The complex biopsychosocial problems associated with maternal substance use present multiple challenges to the successful integration of obstetrical care and treatment services. However, by using a health care approach based on staff collaboration and ongoing communication that ensures patients are treated with dignity and respect, they can receive the care necessary for a healthy pregnancy and a stable recovery.

REFERENCES

Cassidy, B. & Cyna, A. M. (2004). Challenges that opioid-dependent women present to the obstetric anaesthetist. *Anaesthesia and Intensive Care, 32,* 494–501.
Centers for Disease Control. (1989). The Surgeon General's 1989 paper on reducing the health consequences of smoking. *MMWR, 38,* 17–18.

Cherubin, C. E. (1971). Infectious disease problems of narcotic addicts. *Archives of Internal Medicine, 128*, 309–313.

Cherubin, C. E., Baden, M., Kavaler, F., Lerner, S., & Cline, W. (1968). Infective endocarditis in narcotic addicts. *Annals of Internal Medicine, 69*(6), 1091–1098.

Curet, L. B., & Hsi, A. C. (2002). Drug abuse during pregnancy. *Clinical Obstetrics and Gynecology, 45*(1), 73–88.

Finnegan, L. P. (Ed.) (1979). *Drug dependency in pregnancy: clinical management of mother and child.* National Institute on Drug Abuse Services Research Monograph Series. Washington, DC: DHEW Publication No. 79–678.

Finnegan, L. P., Hagan, T., & Kaltenbach, K. (1991). Opioid dependence: scientific foundations for clinical practice, pregnancy and substance abuse: perspectives and directions. *Proceedings of the New York Academy of Medicine, 67*(3), 223–239.

Gordis, E. (1990). Alcohol and women. *Alcohol Alert NIAA, 10*(PH290), 1–4.

Holbrook, A. M., Baxter, J. K., Jones, H. E., Heil, S., Coyle, M., Martin, P., Stine, S., & Kaltenbach, K. (2012). Infections and obstetrical outcomes in opioid-dependent pregnant women maintained on methadone or buprenorphine. *Addiction, 107*(Suppl. 1), 83–90.

Jones, H. E, Berkman, N., Kline, T., Middlesteadt Ellerson, R., Browne, F., Poulton, W., & Wechsberg, W. M. (2011). Initial efficacy of a woman-focused intervention for pregnant African-American women. *International Journal of Pediatrics, 389285*; Epub March 23.

Jones, H. E., Johnson, R. E., & Milio, L. (2006). Post-cesarean pain management of patients maintained on methadone or buprenorphine. *American Journal on Addictions, 15*, 258–9.

Jones, H. E., O'Grady, K. E., Johnson, R. E., Dahne, J., Lemoine, L. I., Milio, L., Ordean, A. & Selby, P. (2009). Management of acute post-partum pain in patients maintained on methadone or buprenorphine during pregnancy. *American Journal of Drug and Alcohol Abuse, 35*, 151–6.

Meyer, M., Paranya, G., Keefer Norris, A., et al. (2010). Intrapartum and postpartum analgesia for women maintained on buprenorphine during pregnancy. *European Journal of Pain, 14*, 939–943.

Naeye, R. L. (1973). Fetal complications of maternal heroin addiction: abnormal growth, infections, and episodes of stress. *Journal of Pediatrics, 83*(6), 1055–1061.

10

Helping Women with Substance Use Disorders Care for Their Drug-Exposed Newborn and Enhance Their Parenting Skills

OVERVIEW

In this chapter we discuss the challenges for both mothers and hospital staff in caring for the newborn who has been prenatally exposed to substances. We describe neonatal abstinence syndrome (NAS) and its treatment regimens. We stress the importance of educating mothers about the medical aspects of NAS, hospital procedures, the need for mothers and infants to room together rather than separately, and staff expectations. We discuss the value of a NAS support group to address maternal feelings of anxiety, guilt, and rejection, and we outline the use of a staff liaison to reduce tensions between mothers and hospital staff. The chapter concludes with a summary that emphasizes key points.

INTRODUCTION

Pregnant women with substance use disorders often need extensive support in caring for their newborn, regardless of previous births and whether or not they have been successful in achieving abstinence. It is presumed that illicit substance use impairs parental functioning, and it certainly may in terms of physical and psychological availability—but the ability to provide nurturing, responsive care is a function of psychological and psychiatric factors that occur within maternal addiction rather than substance use *per se.* Their parenting abilities reflect the complex array of biopsychosocial problems associated with maternal substance use disorders. Thus, they are often children of parents who have used substances and victims of sexual and physical abuse and have comorbid psychiatric illness (see Chapter 5 for a complete discussion of biopsychosocial factors). Pregnant women with substance use disorders need supportive, dyadic-centered newborn services to optimize pregnancy outcomes.

NEONATAL ABSTINENCE SYNDROME

A primary focus for the postpartum woman with an opioid use disorder is whether or not her infant will experience neonatal abstinence syndrome (NAS) and so may require pharmacological treatment. NAS is a term for newborn withdrawal following prenatal exposure to a number of illicit and/or licit drugs. The most severe withdrawal requiring pharmacological treatment is usually associated with opioids and is characterized by signs and symptoms of central nervous system hyperirritability; gastrointestinal irregularities; respiratory distress; and autonomic symptoms (Kaltenbach et al., 1998). A high-pitched cry, a hyperactive Moro reflex, increased muscle tone, sleep disturbances, tremors, and seizures are signs of central nervous system excitation due to NAS. Gastrointestinal effects of NAS include poor feeding, excessive sucking, regurgitation, and diarrhea. Autonomic disturbances include sweating, fever, yawning, sneezing, and mottling, while respiratory dysregulation is indicated by nasal stuffiness and rapid respiration (Finnegan & Kaltenbach, 1992). Most infants prenatally exposed to opioids (e.g., heroin, OxyContin, Percocet, methadone, buprenorphine), will exhibit NAS symptoms, with a high percentage requiring pharmacological intervention.

The severity and presentation of NAS differ based on the specific opioid involved. Withdrawal from heroin may not be as severe as withdrawal from methadone, but untreated heroin use in pregnant women is associated with a high incidence of fetal demise, prematurity, and intrauterine growth restriction (e.g., Glass & Evans, 1972; Kandall et al., 1977). While the incidence of withdrawal requiring treatment is similar for methadone and buprenorphine, the amount of medication needed for treatment and the length of hospital stay are significantly less for buprenorphine-exposed infants compared to methadone-exposed infants (Jones et al., 2010). The withdrawal associated with oxycodone (e.g., Oxycontin, Percocet) may also have unique characteristics, but there have not yet been any studies examining NAS related to this opioid.

Nonopioid drugs can also cause behaviors consistent with withdrawal and/or can exacerbate NAS, notably benzodiazepines, nicotine, selective serotonin reuptake inhibitors (SSRIs), and alcohol. Cocaine and methamphetamines do not cause withdrawal, but infants prenatally exposed to these substances may exhibit behaviors similar to newborns experiencing NAS. With the exception of benzodiazepines, infants usually do not require treatment for prenatal exposure to these drugs. There is evidence that suggests that the withdrawal resulting from opioid and benzodiazepine use is more severe and more difficult to manage than opioid withdrawal alone (Berghella et al., 2003, Seligman et al., 2008). Although the neonatal behavior syndrome associated with SSRI exposure has been found to have self-limiting symptoms that can be managed with supportive care (Moses-Kolko et al., 2005), when SSRIs are used by pregnant women maintained on methadone or buprenorphine, they have been found to exacerbate the length of treatment needed for NAS (Jansson, et al., 2010; Kaltenbach et al., 2012). Prenatal nicotine exposure has also been found to exacerbate the expression of NAS in NAS associated with prenatal opioid exposure (Bakstad et al., 2009; Choo et al., 2004; Jones et al., in press; Winklbaur et al., 2009).

Treatment decisions about the initiation of pharmacotherapy, control of withdrawal, and medication taper are made with the help of an abstinence scoring tool such as the Finnegan score (Finnegan & Kaltenbach, 1992) or a modified Finnegan score such as the MOTHER NAS Measure (Jones et al., 2010).

When pharmacological treatment is required, a medication most commonly used in the United States is morphine sulfate solution (Sarkar & Donn, 2006). If the infant has been exposed to multiple substances, including nonopioids, phenobarbital, in addition to or instead of morphine sulfate, will often be used. The infant receives escalating doses of the medication until the symptoms are under control and then is weaned from the medication. Most infants who require medication will begin NAS treatment within 2 to 3 days after birth. The length of treatment is highly variable and on average ranges from several days to several weeks.

For examples of scoring and treatment protocols, see Finnegan and Kaltenbach (1992), Jansson et al. (2009), and Jones et al. (2010; with supplementary materials available online).

In addition to pharmacological treatment, supportive treatment can be most helpful for infants exhibiting signs of withdrawal. Infants should be kept in a quiet, dimly lit room and should be handled gently. Swaddling helps to moderate the infant's agitation, and providing a pacifier may eliminate the baby's frantic attempts to get his or her fingers into the mouth. Some infants are soothed by rocking. Infants may have their own idiosyncratic responses to different techniques, so caregivers should identify what works best for each infant (Velez & Jansson, 2008).

NAS EDUCATION AND SUPPORT

Pregnant women with substance use disorders are frequently very anxious regarding their infant experiencing NAS. As described in Chapter 9, it is extremely helpful to have a designated staff member serve as a liaison between patient and hospital staff. The staff liaison can reduce their anxiety by ensuring that prenatal services include information on NAS, why and how their infant may receive treatment, and medical staff expectations regarding maternal behaviors during the infant's hospitalization.

A NAS support group facilitated by the staff liaison can be a highly effective mechanism for providing this information within a compassionate, sensitive framework. Such a group can be used to present specific medical information on NAS, including withdrawal due to opioid exposure; other drugs that affect withdrawal, such as benzodiazepines, SSRIs, and nicotine; timing of withdrawal; and symptoms and treatment of withdrawal. It is important for mothers to understand that NAS is a time-limited phenomenon and that for those infants who require treatment, the severity of NAS has not been shown to affect development outcome (Kaltenbach & Finnegan, 1986). In addition, it is important that mothers receiving medication-assisted treatment with methadone or buprenorphine understand that whether or not their infant will need to be treated is not related to which medication they are receiving or their dose. There is no difference between infants born to women maintained on methadone or buprenorphine in terms of the likelihood of requiring pharmacotherapy for NAS (Jones et al., 2010), and there is no relationship between dose and severity of NAS (Cleary et al., 2010; Jones et al., 2005; Lejeune et al., 2006).

Several issues related to NAS can trigger emotional responses from mothers and/or caregivers; these can best be addressed within a support group setting. Two paramount emotional issues associated with NAS are guilt and rejection. Mothers may experience considerable guilt that their infant will undergo withdrawal because of their addiction. Such guilt can be eased with the help of a support group that focuses on understanding how important the mother's commitment to treatment is for the health of her baby; how medication-assisted treatment helps to stabilize the uterine environment of the fetus; and the variability of NAS—some infants of mothers maintained on high doses of methadone or buprenorphine may not require treatment. Support groups that include women who have previously delivered an infant who had NAS can also provide valuable peer support from their personal experiences.

Some NAS symptoms, such as high-pitched cry, poor feeding, hypertonicity, and inconsolability, can cause the mother to believe that she is inadequate and that the infant is rejecting her. Infants with NAS present difficult challenges for even the most skilled caregivers, and the continuous high-pitched cry and irritability can easily make a mother feel like she is not meeting the baby's needs.

Babies with NAS may suck frantically but have difficulty feeding due to ineffective sucking reflexes, leaving mothers discouraged and disconsolate over their inability to meet such a basic need. The hypertonicity exhibited by infants with NAS eliminates any cuddling or molding into a mother's arms and can make the mother feel as if the infant is pushing away from her. Any of these behaviors can hinder mother–child interactions, so mothers must understand that their infant's behavior is not a reaction to their caregiving. Mothers need to be taught soothing techniques of swaddling and rocking; the benefits of using a pacifier to alleviate frantic sucking; the need for a quiet, dimly lit room so as not to overstimulate the infant; methods to assist the infant in feeding; and how to be sensitive to the infant's cues. Additionally, the support group can provide mothers with a forum for expressing their feelings where they can receive appropriate and constructive feedback.

In addition to understanding NAS, mothers must know what to expect and what is expected of them. Every effort must be made to kept mother and infant together in the same room. This "rooming-in" approach is related to fewer babies requiring medication for NAS (Hodgson & Abrahams, 2012). A prenatal visit to the postpartum unit to see the environment and become familiar with the routine can help reduce anxieties, thereby eliminating inappropriate behaviors that may cause tension between mothers and staff. Mothers should be provided with a thorough explanation of NAS scoring, including a review of all the symptoms; the timetable for scoring NAS symptoms (e.g., every 4 hours before feeding), and how decisions are made to treat the infant. Mothers need to clearly understand hospital policies regarding whether they will be allowed to have their baby "room in" or if the baby will be required to stay in the nursery. Specific expectations regarding behavior in the nursery need to be reviewed (e.g., loud talking is not acceptable, infants who are asleep may not be awakened because infants with NAS have difficulty sleeping for prolonged periods, and there must be respect for both staff and nursery rules).

CLINICAL MANAGEMENT

As with the obstetrical team discussed in Chapter 9, nursery staff may exhibit prejudicial and judgmental attitudes toward mothers of infants with NAS. Advocacy and education by a staff liaison may be necessary to eliminate tension between mothers and staff. Nursery staff must have a clear understanding of the benefits of medication-assisted treatment and must show respect for the mother's efforts toward recovery.

Most nurseries today use a family-centered treatment approach that is based on dignity and respect and involves staff collaboration with families, family participation in care, and open communication. However, this may not be the case for mothers with substance use disorders because of mutual negative behaviors by staff and mothers and their partners. The staff liaison can play a critical role in facilitating a family-centered approach. An effective tool for the liaison staff and mother/partner is to meet weekly with nursery staff, social work staff, and physicians (when possible) during the infant's hospitalization so that family and staff can discuss how things are going, identify what's working well and why, and mutually identify strategies to resolve problems.

CLINICAL SERVICES FOR MOTHERS

In addition to the stress of having an infant with NAS, which may require an extended hospital stay, mothers are faced with the ever-present reality that they are being judged, both formally and informally, on their ability to care for their child and may face loss of custody. (See Chapter 1 for a discussion of the federal CAPTA law and individual states' interpretation of child abuse statues that may be used to prosecute women or terminate parental rights.) The treatment program must provide clinical support and appropriate services to help the new mother cope and navigate the multiple systems affecting her life during this vulnerable time. Treatment plans and individual counseling should identify what she needs to do to respond to the needs of her child within the framework of institutional norms and expectations.

SUMMARY

The care of newborn prenatally exposed to substances can be challenging for both mother and staff. The new mother's ability to meet this challenge can be enhanced with education and support about what her infant is undergoing, the medical care the baby will receive, and how she can best parent her infant. NAS is an expected and treatable condition. Rooming-in can be beneficial for mother and infant. Collaborating with the nursery staff and maintaining a dialogue to identify and address any problems that may arise can be very effective in reducing tensions and negative attitudes. In this way, both mother and staff can work together to provide optimal care for the infant.

REFERENCES

Bakstad, B., Sarfi, M., Welle-Strand, G., & Ravndal, E. (2009). Opioid maintenance treatment during pregnancy: Occurrence and severity of neonatal abstinence syndrome. *European Addiction Research, 15,* 128–134.

Berghella, V., Lim, P., Hill, M. K, Cherpes, J., Chennat, J., & Kaltenbach, K. (2003). Maternal methadone dose and neonatal withdrawal. *American Journal of Obstetrics and Gynecology, 189*(2), 312–317.

Choo, R. E., Huestis, M. A., Schroeder, J. R., Shin, A. S., & Jones, H. E. (2004). Neonatal abstinence syndrome in methadone exposed infants is altered by level of prenatal tobacco exposure. *Drug and Alcohol Dependence, 75*, 253–260.

Cleary, B. J., Donnelly, J., Strawbridge, J., Gallagher, P. J., Fahey, T., Clarke, M., & Murphy, D. J. (2010). Methadone dose and neonatal abstinence syndrome: Systematic review and meta-analysis. *Addiction, 105*, 2071–2084.

Finnegan, L. P., & Kaltenbach, K. (1992). The assessment and management of neonatal abstinence syndrome. In Hoekelman, Friedman, Nelson, & Seidel (Eds.), *Primary pediatric care* (3rd ed., pp. 1367–1378). St. Louis, MO: C. V. Mosby Company.

Glass, L., & Evans, H. E. (1972). Narcotic withdrawal in the newborn. *American Family Physician, 6*, 75–78.

Hodgson, Z. G., & Abrahams, R. R. (2012). A rooming-in program to mitigate the need to treat for opiate withdrawal in the newborn. *Journal of Obstetrics and Gynaecology Canada, 34*(5), 475–81.

Jansson, L. M., DiPietro, J. A., Elko, A., & Velez, M. (2010). Autonomic functioning and neonatal abstinence syndrome. *Drug and Alcohol Dependence, 109*, 198–204.

Jansson, L. M., Velez, M., & Harrow, C. (2009). The opioid exposed newborn: assessment and pharmacologic management. *Journal of Opioid Management, 5*, 47–55.

Jones, H. E., Heil, S. H., Tuten, M., Chisolm, M. S., Foster, J. M., O'Grady, K. E., & Kaltenbach, K. (in press). Cigarette smoking in opioid-dependent pregnant women: Neonatal and maternal outcomes. *Drug and Alcohol Dependence.*

Jones, H., Kaltenbach, K., Heil, S., Stine, S., Coyle, M., Arria, A., O'Grady, K., Selby, P., Martin, P., & Fisher, G. (2010). Neonatal abstinence syndrome following methadone or buprenorphine exposure. *New England Journal of Medicine, 363*, 2320–2331.

Jones, H. E., Johnson, R. E., Jasinski, D. R., O'Grady, K. E., Chisholm, C. A., Choo, R. E., Crocetti, M., Dudas, R., Harrow, C., Huestis, M. A., Jansson, L. M., Lantz, M., Lester, B. M., & Milio, L. (2005). Buprenorphine versus methadone in the treatment of pregnant opioid-dependent patients: effects on the neonatal abstinence syndrome. *Drug and Alcohol Dependence, 79*, 1–10.

Kaltenbach, K., Berghella, V., & Finnegan, L. P. (1998). Opioid dependence during pregnancy: Effects and management. *Obstetrics and Gynecology Clinics of North America, 25*(1), 139–151.

Kaltenbach, K., & Finnegan, L. P. (1986). Neonatal abstinence syndrome, pharmacotherapy and developmental outcome. *Neurobehavioral Toxicology and Teratology, 8*, 353–355.

Kaltenbach, K., Holbrook, A., Coyle, M., Heil, S., Salisbury, A.L., Stine, S., Martin, P., & Jones, H. E. (2012). Predicting treatment for neonatal abstinence syndrome in infants born to women maintained on opioid agonist medication. *Addiction, 107*(Suppl. 1), 45–52.

Kandall, S. R., Albin, S., Gartner, L. M., Lee, K. S., Eidelman, J., & Lowinson, J. (1977) The narcotic-dependent mother: fetal and neonatal consequences. *Early Human Development, 1*, 159–169.

Lejeune, C., Simmat-Durand, L., Gourarier, L., Aubisson, S., & Groupe d'Etudes Grossesse et Addictions (2006). Prospective multicenter observational study of 260 infants born to 259 opiate-dependent mothers on methadone or high-dose buprenophine substitution. *Drug and Alcohol Dependence, 82,* 250–257.

Moses-Kolko, E. L., Bogen, D., Bregar, AQ., Levin, B., Perel, J., Uhl, K., & Wisner, K. (2005). Neonatal signs after late in-utero exposure to serotonin reuptake inhibitors: Literature review and implications for clinical applications. *Journal of the American Medical Association, 293,* 2372–2383.

Sarkar, S., & Donn, S. M. (2006). Management of neonatal abstinence syndrome in neonatal intensive care units: a nation survey. *Journal of Perinatology, 26,* 15–17.

Seligman, N., Salva, N., Hayes, E., Dysart, K., Pequignot, E. C., & Baxter, J. K. (2008). Predicting length of treatment for neonatal abstinence syndrome in methadone-exposed neonates. *American Journal of Obstetrics and Gynecology, 199,* 396.e1–396.e7.

Velez, M., & Jansson, L. (2008). The opioid dependent mother and newborn dyad: nonpharmacologic care. *Journal of Addiction Medicine, 2*(3), 113–120.

Winklbaur, B., Baewert, A., Jagsch, R., Rohrmeister, K., Metz, V., Aeschbach Jachmann, C., Thau, K., & Fischer, G. (2009). Association between prenatal tobacco exposure and outcome of neonates born to opioid-maintained mothers: Implications for treatment. *European Addiction Research, 15,* 150–156.

11

Components of a Comprehensive Substance Use Treatment Program for Pregnant Women

OVERVIEW

C hapter 11 weaves together the multiple components and aspects of care discussed in the preceding chapters. In this chapter we discuss the specific aspects of a comprehensive substance use treatment program for pregnant women. To be effective, such a program must address each domain of a pregnant patient's life that may be compromised by substance use: survival, physical health, psychological health, relationship health, social functioning, economic independence, and child-centered services, in addition to program-wide functions cutting across all of these domains. Within each domain, we summarize the content areas to be covered and offer practical tips for covering these topics. When used appropriately, objective methods for verifying drug abstinence are an important component of comprehensive treatment. We give examples of measures that can be used for this purpose and how the results can be used to plan or focus treatment services. Further, because relapse to substance use is often a part of the complete recovery process, we suggest ways to address this issue, both before and after it happens. Finally, a summary with take-home messages from the chapter is provided.

INTRODUCTION

As discussed in this book's introduction, the political and social issues of the 1970s and 1980s brought into focus the unique issues related to women's health. As a result of these converging forces, programs to treat substance use disorders were remodeled or created to better serve women. During this time of social change, awareness grew regarding the social factors that shape women's lives, and researchers studied how women's substance use differs from that of men. Women's experience of substance use was found to be shaped by gender, race/ethnicity, sexual preferences, social class, culture of community and country, and morality, reproduction, and parenting inequalities between men and women (Finkelstein et al., 1993). An often-ignored force that influences women's lives is the role of personal religious beliefs and religious viewpoints in the culture itself.

Women-centered programs to treat substance use disorders were established to address the unique needs of women who use legal and illegal drugs. Many of these programs have been shown to improve the maternal and neonatal outcomes of patients treated during pregnancy (see the book's introduction for a summary of this literature). The literature shows generally high agreement about the components that should be a part of such women-centered treatment programming. These domains are survival, physical health, psychological health, relationship health, social functioning, economic independence, and child-centered services, in addition to program-wide functions cutting across all of these domains. Table 11.1 summarizes these domains and the relevant components of care within each one that have been found to be aspects of a successful and comprehensive treatment program for substance-using women. There is general agreement in the literature about the types of topics that should be covered (e.g., Brotman et al., 1985; Chavkin, 1991; Finkelstein et al., 1993; Finnegan, 1991; Finnegan et al., 1991; Hutchins & Alexander, 1990; Jessup, 1990; Jones et al., 1999, 2006; Kaltenbach & Finnegan, 1998; Kumpfer, 1991; Reed, 1987; Suffet & Brotman, 1984).

SPECIFIC CONTENT TO BE COVERED
DURING TREATMENT

Seven of the eight domains represent specific aspects of a patient's recovery and are discussed in terms of the explicit treatment-oriented content that could be a part of care in this domain. The eighth domain deals with program-wide functions cutting across all of these domains.

Survival

Unless a patient's basic survival needs (food, clothing, housing, and safety) are quickly addressed, cessation of substance use can be severely impeded (Finnegan et al., 1991) because basic survival will always come before higher-order needs.

Having a small food bank supplied by donations from grocery stores, discount stores, and local community and religious organizations can be a jumpstart to building trust and establishing a caring relationship with patients. At the very least, being able to provide patients with a current list of local food banks, places that supply meals to homeless individuals, and instructions about how to sign up for government-assisted food programs can be helpful (see Chapter 6 for more details). Following up with patients about the adequacy of their nutrition and success in signing up for food programs is important, as they may need continued assistance navigating the bureaucratic systems to receive food. Although in-depth discussions of the relationship between nutrition and recovery can wait until patients are stabilized in treatment, the importance of eating healthy foods (e.g., fruits and vegetables, fiber, whole grains) rather than processed foods and the need for adequate hydration should be stressed early on. Many patients drink very little unless it is a soft drink or other sugar-filled beverage. The importance of drinking water and avoiding drinks with high sugar content should be emphasized to support health maintenance.

Clothing needs for pregnant women are ongoing, given their advancing gestation. Maintaining a clothing closet can be of great help to patients. A rotating set of staff can be assigned to contact and solicit donations of used or unsold maternity clothing from individuals in the community and community businesses and organizations (e.g., dry-cleaning businesses with abandoned clothes, houses of worship, Goodwill, clothing stores, etc.). This will keep a continuing supply of clothes that change with the seasons available to patients. Some patients resist wearing maternity clothes as part of their avoidance or denial process regarding their pregnancy. Helping patients to select clothing choices that are flattering to them in a nonsexual way can be a sensitive yet important issue for their recovery.

Clothes for patients' children may also be needed. Many patients have at least one child and on average have two children (e.g., Kissin et al., 2001), and these children often need clothing and footwear appropriate for the season. Keeping donations on hand at the clinic can help patients meet their families' needs.

With both the food bank and the clothing closets for women and children, there need to be clearly established rules regarding the number of items and the frequency of clothing bank visits that patients are allowed for themselves and their children. Only one patient should be allowed in the clothing closet at a time. To avoid disagreements over who gets what clothing, having prefilled opaque bags labeled by size (and gender for children) can help reduce staff and patient conflicts or conflicts between patients. Any items that are not taken within a month of their arrival to the program should be donated to another organization or discarded.

Table 11-1. COMPONENTS OF A COMPREHENSIVE TREATMENT

DOMAIN	TREATMENT SERVICE				
Program-wide functions cutting across all categories	Advocacy	Assessment	Case management	Community-based services	Community education and linkages
Survival	Food	Clothing	Housing	Transportation	Physical safety from abuser
Physical health	Medical care (prenatal, obstetrical, pediatric, general, dental)	Medical stabili-zation services	Pharmacological services	HIV counseling and testing	Lamaze class
Psychological health	Components to build self-esteem	Trauma recovery	Mental health services	Pharmacological services	
Relationship health	Relationship-building skills		Life skills	Trauma recovery	Parenting services: skills train-ing and support
Social functioning	Assertiveness training	Legal services	Life skills	Trauma recovery	
Economic independence	Education Vocational training and assistance	Legal services	Life skills	Job acquisition and mainte-nance skills	
Child-centered services	Child care during treatment	Child develop-ment services	Child protec-tion and welfare services	Foster care recruitment, training, and support	Newborn caregiving

PROGRAM FOR SUBSTANCE USE DISORDERS DURING PREGNANCY

Coordination and collaboration	Crisis intervention	Culturally specific staff and services	Follow-up Aftercare services	Home visiting and other in-home services	Multidisciplinary assessment and treatment teams	Outreach
Obstetrical education	Nutritional counseling	Relapse prevention		HIV risk behavior reduction skills	Drug, alcohol and tobacco education	Counseling (Individual, Group & Family)
		Relapse prevention	Skills building	HIV risk behavior reduction skills	Drug, alcohol and tobacco education	Counseling (Individual, Group & Family)
			Skills building	HIV risk behavior reduction skills		Counseling (Individual, Group & Family)
			Skills building			
			Skills building			
Children's treatment services						

Safe and stable housing is likely the most formidable survival challenge patients face and is a contributing factor to poor treatment outcomes (Hagan et al., 1994; Tuten et al., 2003). For programs that cannot afford to hire a case manager, enlisting a member of the clinic staff to maintain a list of housing resources is one way to help staff and patients stay on top of the ever-changing regulations and resources for housing. Regularly asking patients about their housing is necessary as housing stability is often fragile in this population. Moreover, many transitional housing facilities or shelters may not allow children or more than a specific number of children to live in the building. In addition, there can be restrictions (sometimes illegal) on the type and/or amount of medication women may have on the property. Women receiving medication-assisted treatment (i.e., methadone or buprenorphine) often face discriminatory practices when seeking temporary housing. In addition, transitional houses or recovery houses are often unwilling to take women (pregnant or not) and children due to liability issues. A point person from the clinic can be designated to establish and maintain connections with these organizations and to facilitate the relationships between women and the housing manager.

Some women living in unsafe or marginal housing situations may be reluctant to move to more formalized and structured living due to fears about leaving their partner, rigidity of rules, loss of freedom, etc. Discussing the specific barriers and fears they have about any new living arrangements, as well as giving them a tour (in person or with pictures or videos), can alleviate the fear of the unknown and bolster their motivation to enter housing. Using a behavioral contract (see Chapter 6 for an example) to have the patient try the housing for two nights can be a "foot in the door" approach for helping her to sample the housing and its benefits. Once the two nights are completed, the patient can sign a new behavioral contract agreeing to live in the housing for a longer period. The time period should be negotiated with the patient. While a short-term contract is beneficial for having patients sample this housing, the ultimate goal is to have patients agree to a more extended period living in safe housing.

Due to the deprivation in which many of these women grow up and continue to live in, only a few patients treated for substance use disorders during pregnancy have a valid driver's license. Even if they do have a license, they often do not have access to a vehicle and thus depend on others or the public transportation system. Lack of transportation can be a serious barrier to attending both treatment and the other appointments that are part of a full recovery. Programs that provide transportation assistance (e.g., a car or van service to pick patients up) have been shown to be more effective in improving outpatient treatment retention than vouchers or tokens for public transportation (Friedmann et al., 2001). This may be due to the additional structure and informal social support the program-supported transportation provides (Friedmann et al., 2001), and these structured forms of transportation can be a key to increasing the likelihood that patients will access treatment and other appointments.

Educating patients about domestic violence and protecting them from abusive partners are discussed in Chapter 12.

Physical Health

There is a relatively large body of evidence supporting the relationship between adequate prenatal care and improved delivery and neonatal outcomes of pregnant women with substance use disorders (e.g., Armstrong et al., 2003; El-Mohandes et al., 2003). These studies suggest that, in general, the first priority for medical care is prenatal care. A detailed discussion of prenatal care is provided in Chapter 9.

General medical care for the pregnant patient with a substance use disorder is also important and is often provided as part of obstetrical and prenatal care. Aspects of general medical care that would be expected to be evaluated would be HIV, hepatitis, sexually transmitted diseases, diabetes, hypertension, and other common co-occurring medical conditions.

Medical stabilization services include medication-assisted withdrawal (see Chapter 7) and opioid agonist maintenance for opioid dependence (see Chapter 6). Methadone maintenance is the standard of treatment for opioid-dependent pregnant women. However, recent research suggests that buprenorphine may also be considered a first-line option for pregnant women who are new to opioid agonist treatment or are already maintained on buprenorphine (Jones et al., 2010). Two Treatment Improvement Protocols, TIP #40 and #43, provide details about the assessment, induction, and maintenance of pregnant patients on methadone or buprenorphine (Center for Substance Abuse Treatment, 2004, 2005).

Like any medications given during pregnancy, methadone and buprenorphine have associated risks or side effects for both mother and child. The risks for the mother are the same as for nonpregnant patients. The status of a patient's pregnancy can introduce additional complications and considerations. For example, reductions in fetal heart rate and fetal movement have been observed after methadone dosing. The implications of these fetal changes on short-term or long-term growth and development are unknown. There is also the risk of neonatal withdrawal (e.g., poor feeding, disrupted sleep, extreme irritability, tremors, etc.) following *in utero* exposure to opioid agonists (see Chapter 10). Scoring tools are available to assess and guide medication treatment regimens for neonatal withdrawal. The benefits of opioid agonist treatment over continued illicit opioid use during pregnancy include eliminating the exposure to illicit opioid use; decreasing the incidence of HIV risk behaviors associated with illicit substance use; reducing the frequency of drug-seeking behaviors, including exchanging sex for drugs; protecting the fetus from repeated episodes of opioid withdrawal; and promoting retention in treatment (see Jones et al., 1999, and Kaltenbach & Finnegan, 1998, for reviews).

Buprenorphine is being prescribed frequently to pregnant patients in treatment for opioid dependence. Currently available data about prenatal exposure to buprenorphine (in the form of Subutex) do not indicate that it is associated with greater risk to the mother or embryo/fetus than methadone (Jones et al., 2010). However, the management of patients taking buprenorphine presents unique challenges and potential benefits compared to methadone (Jones, Finnegan, & Kaltenbach, 2012). The two medications work differently and cannot be used interchangeably.

Naltrexone, a medication originally developed to treat heroin overdose, has been available for the treatment of opioid dependence for almost 30 years, and for the treatment of alcohol dependence for almost 10 years. In contrast to opioid agonists such as methadone and buprenorphine, naltrexone is an opioid antagonist. Until the recent development of long-acting injectable and implant formulations of the drug (e.g., Vivitrol), its use for the treatment of either disorder has been quite limited in practice. The long-acting formulations have spurred increased interest in its use for the treatment of both disorders. Although it has not been approved for the treatment of opioid dependence in pregnant women, it is almost certain that providers of services to these two populations will prescribe this medication to nonpregnant women in treatment for substance use who will subsequently become pregnant. There is no available research that can guide providers in how best to respond in this situation. There is no protocol for medication-assisted withdrawal for these women. There is insufficient research examining subtle teratologic effects associated with *in utero* exposure to naltrexone. Likewise, research on breast milk concentrations of naltrexone and its impact on the neonate is lacking. Finally, relapse to illicit opioid use in pregnant women receiving naltrexone treatment may pose a significant danger to both the woman and her fetus that is not present for pregnant women receiving opioid agonist treatment, because they would be exposed to a bolus of an opioid without the buffering effect of previous opioid agonist medication. This latter concern suggests that any pregnant woman maintained on naltrexone be closely monitored for medication compliance to minimize this risk (Jones et al., 2012).

As discussed in Chapter 8, many patients treated for substance use disorders during pregnancy have co-occurring psychiatric disorders for which medications may be needed. These medications may be in addition to other medications needed to treat general or obstetrical issues. Many of the women who seek treatment for substance use disorders during pregnancy have very limited financial resources and are thus likely to need help to pay for medications. Staff should be aware of the local or commercial resources (e.g., some pharmaceutical companies have programs for indigent populations that offer medications for free or at least at cost) to help patients obtain needed pharmacological treatment.

Treatment for substance use disorders during pregnancy represents an optimal time for providing HIV prevention services (Malow et al., 2006) as well as regular testing. Testing should be performed both initially at intake and then close to the time of delivery, provided at least a month has passed since intake testing.

Chapter 9 discusses obstetrical education, nutritional counseling, and more general health education that may also be a part of this treatment element.

Psychological Health

Although patients have first-hand experience with substances of abuse, they often lack accurate information about them, their effects, and their health consequences to mother and fetus. For example, dispelling the myth that "hard drugs" are worse for mother and fetus than "legal" drugs like alcohol and nicotine can be vital, particularly given the extremely deleterious effects associated with alcohol (physical and brain problems) and cigarette smoking (low birth weight and prematurity) (Jones et al., in press).

There are some excellent evidence-based treatments for empowering women to reduce their HIV risks. For example, a woman-focused intervention showed significant reductions in daily alcohol and cocaine use and less victimization than did a matched control condition (Wechsberg et al., 2006). A modified version of this intervention also showed some efficacy in pregnant women who have a substance use disorder (Jones et al., 2011).

Counseling that covers the diverse aspects of recovery in multiple areas of life functioning has been a part of many comprehensive care programs (e.g., Jansson et al., 1996). In both individual and group counseling, similar topics should be covered (e.g., relapse prevention, relationship building, and assertive communication). Examples of specific topics are discussed below. The individual counseling sessions allow patients to focus on their recovery and discuss their personal situation with the counselor. Group therapy will reinforce the material provided in individual counseling by allowing patients to provide and exchange information with the help of the counselor and to practice their skills in role-plays. Family counseling can take the form of an educational group where the family members of patients can receive education; in some cases they, too, can also recover from substance use. Family members who do not use substances can learn how to support the patient in abstinence.

Chapter 12 discusses trauma recovery in pregnant patients.

Art therapy can be a positive addition to the treatment plan (Holt & Kaiser, 2009), especially for patients who have experienced violence and/or victimization (Glover, 1999).

Chapter 8 discusses the treatment of co-occurring psychiatric disorders such as mood and anxiety disorders (e.g., depression, posttraumatic stress disorder) in pregnant patients with substance use disorders. At a minimum, patients should be screened for Axis I and Axis II disorders and should always be rescreened for postpartum depression. Patients with positive screens should receive referrals for evaluation by a psychiatrist.

Numerous manuals provide general or women-specific skills-building exercises (e.g., relapse prevention, stress management, anger management). For example, the manual *Trauma Recovery and Empowerment* (Harris, 1998) has modules aimed at building self-esteem and intimacy and trust, communication, and decision making. Another manual that is well known in the substance use treatment community but is not tailored to pregnant women is *Overcoming Your Alcohol or Drug Problem* (Daley & Marlatt, 2006). This manual has a patient workbook to accompany it and has helpful modules on goal planning, managing cravings, managing thoughts of using substances, managing emotions, and building a support network. The Substance Abuse and Mental Health Services Administration has also published a workbook on anger management for patients with substance use disorders (Reilly et al., 2002). Life skills may include how to use the library, finding drug-free recreational activities in the community, and how to shop for nutritional foods in the grocery store or farmer's market. Patients may need to learn about and practice managing money and working with a household budget.

Relationship Health

Women tend to be relational by nature and define themselves in relation to others. Thus, for the pregnant patient much thought and focus of her treatment may be spent dealing with the relationships she has lost or damaged or will need to create. For example, understanding the patterns and roles that developed in response to parental or caregiver substance use as well as any physical, emotional, and/or sexual abuse and victimization the patient experienced as a child will help the provider in reshaping the patient's behavior (Finkelstein, 1994). Attention should also be given to helping the patient develop healthy relationships with men that are not based primarily on sexual activities but on mutually nurturing and empowering interactions.

As a pregnant woman, the patient has the promise of a new relationship with her unborn child. This maternal role can also be a source of great anxiety, fear, and guilt (Finnegan, 1978; Mackie-Ramos & Rice, 1988). Giving mothers the skills needed to address problem behaviors in their children and also to cope with negative emotions related to their life experiences may be useful to help prevent relapse, as well as to establish positive relationships with their children.

A family therapy group could complement the individual family therapy a patient is participating in and could help the patient work on establishing and repairing relationships, as appropriate.

Social Functioning

Many of these patients need legal services or assistance. They may enter treatment as a result of legal problems or may be facing legal problems such as arrests for drug possession or sale or commercial sex work; less frequent are assault or robbery charges. Providers should have established relationships with the *pro bono* law groups in the area as well as local law schools. These institutions can be good sources of free legal help for patients.

The other common legal issue that patients face is child custody, either of their older children or the new baby. Providers should have good working relationships with the local child protection services to help patients advocate for themselves and to increase the probability that the patient will be treated fairly in this system.

Economic Independence

The need for economic independence cannot be overstated for this patient population. There are several avenues for patients to achieve this level of functioning. One way is by learning a vocation as part of the treatment program. Another is by earning a degree needed to acquire a job, such as a GED. Online versions of GED programs can be taken over a period of months, and computers in the clinic could be set up for this purpose. At a minimum, the treatment program should provide referrals for education in the form of a GED classes or training for a specific vocation.

Once patients have decided on the type of job they would like to have, then they need the tools to apply for a position and obtain it. They need to learn to write a résumé, complete job applications, interview for a job, and negotiate benefits. Several manuals can assist patients with these activities (e.g., Hall et al., 1991). One issue that can be a challenge is that maternity leave is often not paid or even available for women in low-level jobs. The Family and Medical Leave Act (FMLA; U.S. Department of Labor: http://www.dol.gov/whd/fmla/) requires all employers with 50 or more employees within a 75-mile radius to provide *unpaid* leave. FMLA provides for (1) pregnancy leave, (2) parental leave, and (3) intermittent parental leave. Pregnancy leave occurs before the birth of the child and usually requires a health care professional's determination that leave is necessary due to serious complications associated with the pregnancy. Parental leave occurs following the birth of the child, and employers are required to provide a period of parental leave to both mother and father, upon application. However, employees must have been employed for 1 year and worked 1,250 hours before they become eligible. Therefore, any woman hired during pregnancy would not be eligible. The treatment provider, if given permission to speak with the employer, can often help negotiate the time off and return to work after the baby is older.

Many patients being treated for substance use disorders have no financial resources, distrust banks, and use expensive check-cashing establishments to cash their public assistance checks and pay their bills. Staff should identify banks willing to allow customers to maintain checking accounts with very low balances and should help patients to develop a budget and manage money; these skills are key to achieving economic independence. If the woman's partner or family controls the public assistance she receives, helping to empower her to take control of her money is an important element in recovery.

Child-Centered Services

Chapter 5 offers more information on this domain.

One barrier to women seeking and engaging in treatment is the issue of child care. Ideally, child care should be located on site in the program. Having child care on site reduces the burden women may have in finding safe care for their children and the need to drop off the children before coming to the program. Another advantage of having on-site child care is that it allows providers to see first hand the interaction of mother and child and observe the child for any signs that screening for services or interventions might be needed.

The vast majority of programs do not have child development and treatment services on site. Providers should be familiar with the local institutions or organizations that provide pediatric testing, diagnosis, and treatment for behavioral disorders and medical issues. Staff must maintain communication with these outside treatment providers to ensure that they are educated about and sensitive to the special issues that patients and their children may have (e.g., delay in motor and cognitive developmental milestones; interpersonal trauma exposure of mother and/or child).

Staff should also be familiar with and have established relations with local hospitals and their obstetrical, labor and delivery, and postpartum units so that they can provide education about the illness of substance use disorders in women and help reduce the negative attitudes that many providers have about working with these patients. For women who are treated with opioid agonists (methadone or buprenorphine), who used opioids during pregnancy, and/or who have used benzodiazepines, neonatal abstinence syndrome may be an issue (see Chapter 10).

OBJECTIVE METHODS FOR VERIFYING DRUG ABSTINENCE

Regular and objective verification of drug abstinence is an important component of comprehensive treatment for substance use disorders in pregnant women. Many types of biological tests can be used to detect substance use in patients. Two of the most common biological matrices for detecting drugs are urine and saliva. The advantages of saliva testing over urine testing include that a saliva test is a noninvasive method and the collection of saliva can be observed without embarrassment to the patient. A second advantage of saliva testing is that there is a reduced chance of sample adulteration compared to urine samples, because the entire sample collection procedure can be supervised. The disadvantages of saliva drug testing include the small specimen volumes, which restrict the number of analyses that can be performed. There is also the opportunity for contaminating the mouth, either deliberately (e.g., placing a penny in the mouth) or inadvertently. Samples may be difficult to collect from individuals abusing stimulants such as amphetamines and Ecstasy, which cause dry mouth (http://www.toxlab.co.uk/DrugsAbuseScreen.html). It is important to have a good working relationship with a local laboratory that performs urine and saliva testing so that questions about tests can be answered.

An appropriate response to a lapse back to substance use is important because it can help to prevent it from turning into a full-blown relapse. While there are typical warning signs (see Chapter 6) that a lapse may be coming, each patient may have unique signs that should be explored based on her past behavior. The best way to prevent relapse is to recognize the patient's warning signs before substance use occurs; to use ongoing assessment of important psychosocial and psychiatric indicators; to monitor urine drug screens regularly in order to identify initial substance use; and to put interventions into place to prevent a full relapse. The patient's clinical presentation at each visit should be noted for changes that suggest precursors to relapse (e.g., late to appointments, missing appointments, not participating in recreational activities, seeing drug-using friends, giving vague answers about outside-of-treatment activities, avoiding her children). Careful observation and probing questions about the patient's behavior will often reveal what behaviors need to be in place to support drug abstinence (see the case example provided in Chapter 6).

The workbook by Daley and Marlatt (2006) has excellent worksheets and plans for addressing and managing relapse.

SUMMARY

Treatment of substance use disorders in pregnant patients is complex and multifaceted. Programs should address survival needs, physical health (obstetrical and general), psychological health, relationship health, social functioning, economic independence, and services to support the mother and child.

REFERENCES

Armstrong, M. A., Gonzales Osejo, V., Lieberman, L., Carpenter, D. M., Pantoja, P. M., & Escobar, G. J. (2003). Perinatal substance abuse intervention in obstetric clinics decreases adverse neonatal outcomes. *Journal of Perinatology, 23*(1), 3–9.

Brotman, R., Hutson, D., & Suffet, F. (1985). *Pregnant addicts and their children: A comprehensive care approach.* New York: Center for Comprehensive Health Practice, New York Medical College.

Center for Substance Abuse Treatment. (2004). *Clinical guidelines for the use of buprenorphine in the treatment of opioid addiction.* Treatment Improvement Protocol (TIP) Series 40. DHHS Publication No. (SMA) 04-3939. Rockville, MD: Substance Abuse and Mental Health Services Administration.

Center for Substance Abuse Treatment. (2005). *Medication-assisted treatment for opioid addiction in opioid treatment programs.* Treatment Improvement Protocol (TIP) Series 43. DHHS Publication No. (SMA) 05-4048. Rockville, MD: Substance Abuse and Mental Health Services Administration.

Chavkin, W. (1991). Mandatory treatment for drug use during pregnancy. *Journal of the American Medical Association, 266*(11), 1556–1561.

Daley, D. C., & Marlatt, G. A. (2006). *Overcoming your alcohol or drug problem: effective recovery strategies* (2nd ed.). New York: Oxford University Press.

El-Mohandes, A., Herman, A. A., Nabil, El-Khorazaty, M., Katta, P. S., White, D., & Grylack, L. (2003). Prenatal care reduces the impact of illicit drug use on perinatal outcomes. *Journal of Perinatology, 23*(5), 354–360.

Finkelstein, N. (1993). Treatment programming for alcohol and drug-dependent pregnant women. *International Journal of Addictions, 28*(13), 1275–1309.

Finkelstein, N. (1994). Treatment issues for alcohol- and drug-dependent pregnant and parenting women. *Health and Social Work, 19*(1), 7–15.

Finnegan, L. P. (1978). Management of pregnant drug-dependent women. *Annals of the New York Academy of Sciences, 311*, 135–146.

Finnegan, L. P. (1991). Treatment issues for opioid-dependent women during the perinatal period. *Journal of Psychoactive Drugs, 23*(2), 191–201.

Finnegan, L. P., Hagan, T., & Kaltenbach, K. A. (1991). Scientific foundation of clinical practice: Opiate use in pregnant women. *Academy of Medicine, 67*(3), 223–239.

Friedmann, P., Lemon, S. C., & Stein, M. D. (2001). Transportation and retention in outpatient drug abuse treatment programs. *Journal of Substance Abuse Treatment, 21*, 97–103.

Glover, N. M. (1999). Play therapy and art therapy for substance abuse clients who have a history of incest victimization. *Journal of Substance Abuse Treatment, 16*(4), 281–287.

Hagan, T. A., Finnegan, L. P., & Nelson-Zlupko, L. (1994). Impediments to comprehensive models for substance dependent women: Treatment and research questions. *Journal of Psychoactive Drugs, 26*, 163–171.

Hall, S. M., Wasserman, D. A., & Havassy, B. E. (1991). Relapse prevention. *NIDA Research Monograph, 106*, 279–292.

Harris, M. (1998). *Trauma recovery and empowerment: A clinician's guide for working with women in groups.* New York: The Free Press.

Holt, E., & Kaiser, D. H. (2009). The First Step Series: Art therapy for early substance abuse treatment. *The Arts in Psychotherapy, 36*(4), 245–250.

Hutchins, E., & Alexander, G. (1990). *Substance use during pregnancy and its effects on the infant: A review of issues* (HHS Region 11, Perinatal Information Consortium Technical Report Series 90–101). Baltimore: Johns Hopkins University, Department of Maternal and Child Health.

Jansson, L. M., Svikis, D., Lee, J., Paluzzi, P., Rutigliano, P., & Hackerman, F. (1996). Pregnancy and addiction: A comprehensive care model. *Journal of Substance Abuse Treatment, 13*(4), 321–329.

Jessup, M. (1990). The treatment of perinatal addiction: Identification, intervention and advocacy. *Western Journal of Medicine, 152*, 553–558.

Jones, H. E., Berkman, N. D., Kline, T. L., Ellerson, R. M., Browne, F. A., Poulton, W., & Wechsberg, W. M. (2011). Initial feasibility of a woman-focused intervention for pregnant African-American women. *International Journal of Pediatrics,* Epub March 23.

Jones, H. E., Chisolm, M. S., Jansson, L. M., & Terplan, M. (2012). Naltrexone in the treatment of opioid-dependent pregnant women: The case for a considered and measured approach to research. *Addiction,* DOI: 10.1111/j.1360-0443.2012.03811.x [E-pub ahead of print].

Jones, H. E., Finnegan, L. P., & Kaltenbach, K. (2012). Methadone and buprenorphine for the management of opioid dependence in pregnancy. *Drugs, 72*(6), 747–757.

Jones, H. E., Kaltenbach, K., Heil, S. H., Stine, S. M., Coyle, M. G., Arria, A. M., O'Grady, K. E., Selby, P., Martin, P. R., & Fischer, G. (2010). Neonatal abstinence syndrome after methadone or buprenorphine exposure. *New England Journal of Medicine, 363*(24), 2320–2331.

Jones, H. E., Tuten, M., Keyser-Marcus, L., & Svikis, D. S. (2006). Specialty treatment for women. In: E. C. Strain & M. Stitzer (Eds.), *The treatment of opioid dependence* (pp. 455–484). Baltimore, MD: Johns Hopkins University Press.

Jones, H. E., Velez, M. L., McCaul, M. E., & Svikis, D. S. (1999). Special treatment issues for women. In: E. C. Strain & M. Stitzer (Eds.), *Methadone treatment for opioid dependence* (pp. 251–280). Baltimore, MD: Johns Hopkins University Press.

Kaltenbach, K., & Finnegan, L. (1998). Prevention and treatment issues for pregnant cocaine-dependent women and their infants. *Annals of the New York Academy of Sciences, 846*, 329–334.

Kissin, W. B., Svikis, D. S., Morgan, G. D., & Haug, N. A. (2001). Characterizing pregnant drug-dependent women in treatment and their children. *Journal of Substance Abuse Treatment, 21*(1), 27–34.

Kumpfer, K. L. (1991). Treatment programs for drug abusing women. *Future of Children, 1*(1), 50–59.

Mackie-Ramos, R. L., & Rice, J. M. (1988). Group psychotherapy with methadone-maintained pregnant women. *Journal of Substance Abuse Treatment, 5*(3), 151–161.

Malow, R. M., Dévieux, J. G., Rosenberg, R., Dyer, J. G., & Lawrence J. S. (2006). Integrated HIV care: HIV risk outcomes of pregnant substance abusers. *Substance Use & Misuse, 41*(13), 1745–1767.

Reed, B. G. (1987). Developing women-sensitive drug dependence treatment services: Why so difficult? *Journal of Psychoactive Drugs, 19*(2), 151–164.

Reilly, P. M., Shopshire, M. S., Durazzo, T. C., & Campbell, T. A. (2002). *Anger management for substance abuse and mental health clients.* Rockville MD: Center for Substance Abuse Treatment.

Suffet, F., & Brotman, R. A. (1984). Comprehensive care program for pregnant addicts: Obstetrical, neonatal, and child development outcomes. *International Journal of Addictions, 19*(2), 199–219.

Tuten, M., Jones, H. E., & Svikis, D. S. (2003). Comparing homeless and domiciled pregnant substance dependent women on psychosocial characteristics and treatment outcomes. *Drug & Alcohol Dependency, 69*, 95–99.

U.S. Department of Labor, Wage and Hour Division. Available online: http://www.dol.gov/compliance/laws/comp-fmla.htm#overview (accessed November 6, 2012).

Wechsberg, W. M., Luseno, W. K., Lam, W. K., Parry, C. D., & Morojele, N. K. (2006). Substance use, sexual risk, and violence: HIV prevention intervention with sex workers in Pretoria. *AIDS and Behavior, 10*(2), 131–137.

Trauma-Informed Treatment

OVERVIEW

In this chapter we discuss the extremely high prevalence of trauma in women with substance use disorders and the need for services to be trauma-informed. We distinguish between "trauma-informed services" and "trauma-specific services." The discussion includes practical examples, assessments, and manualized, evidence-based models used to treat sequelae of trauma due to abuse or violence. "Trauma" is used as an umbrella term to include the emotional, physical, and sexual abuse that women may have experienced or witnessed. A summary of the chapter presents key points.

INTRODUCTION

As noted in Chapter 5, women with substance use disorders often have a significant history of trauma, with many suffering from posttraumatic stress disorder (PTSD). In one of the first studies that examined addiction and trauma, Covington and Kohen (1984) found that 74% of women with substance use disorders reported a history of sexual abuse, 52% reported physical abuse, and 72% reported emotional abuse. Further studies have supported and expanded on these findings: women in treatment for substance use disorders report a high incidence of domestic violence and physical and sexual abuse as children and as adults (Comfort & Kaltenbach, 1999; Teusch, 1997, Velez et al., 2006). Najavits et al. (1997) found that among women with substance use disorders, 30% to 59% also experience PTSD, typically as a result of childhood physical or sexual abuse. A review of the characteristics of 2,729 women enrolled in treatment programs designed to integrate trauma-informed services with services for co-occurring substance use and mental health disorders found that approximately 75% of these women experienced multiple and repeated abuses, including sexual abuse, physical abuse, and emotional abuse and neglect. The average age of initial sexual and physical abuse was 13 years of age, while the age of onset for emotional and physical neglect was 9 years of age (Becker et al., 2005). Such a pervasive history of trauma has significant implications for health service delivery practices on several levels.

TREATMENT ENVIRONMENT

First is the importance of providing a safe, healing environment. Women must feel safe in the treatment environment, both physically and emotionally. The facility should be in a safe neighborhood and patients should be able to view it as a safe haven, where they can be protected from abusive partners. Women must know that sexual harassment or abuse is not tolerated, and they must feel that they are safe to report it without any repercussions or retribution. They should understand that rules are in place not just to impose restrictions but to ensure the safety of all. These cautions may be especially salient in an environment that serves both men and women but should not be taken for granted in women-only programs.

TRAUMA-INFORMED SERVICES

The recognition that most patients receiving treatment for a substance use disorder have a history of trauma has led to a paradigm shift in treatment, especially in the treatment of women. Behavioral health systems throughout the country have come to recognize that to address the needs of this vulnerable population, the service delivery system must integrate knowledge about trauma, violence, and substance use into systems of care, better known as trauma-informed services. These efforts are reflected in and supported by the National Center for Trauma Informed Care, a technical assistance center within the Substance Abuse Mental Health Services Administration, DHHS (Substance Abuse Mental Health Services Administration, DHHS, 2012).

To be "trauma-informed" means (1) understanding the role that violence and victimization play in the lives of women seeking substance use and mental health services; (2) designing a service system to accommodate the vulnerabilities of trauma survivors; and (3) delivering services in a manner that will facilitate participation in treatment (Harris & Fallot, 2001). This definition touches on several of the elements that need to be included in a trauma-informed system of care. Programs should include a trauma policy or position statement within their policies and procedures to formalize their commitment to providing trauma-informed services. The policies and services must reflect a respect for culture, race, ethnicity, gender, age, sexual orientation, and physical disability.

There should be specific trauma-related practice guidelines and treatment approaches, including procedures to avoid retraumatization. Program staff, including nonclinical staff, need to have specialized training related to trauma so that they are sensitive to the vulnerabilities of trauma survivors, with trauma-informed competencies included in their job standards. Programs need to ensure that the experiences and perspectives of trauma survivors are represented in the development and implementation of services, and specialized trauma programs need to be integrated within mental health and substance use services (Blanch, 2003).

ASSESSMENT

Treatment settings do not routinely assess women for trauma or PTSD. For those programs that do address trauma issues, patients typically perceive the message that they have to be progressing in their recovery before PTSD can be addressed (Morrissey et al., 2005). However, research suggests that trauma-related issues can be addressed concomitantly with substance use treatment without precipitating adverse events (Killeen et al., 2008). Trauma can be evaluated with a clinical assessment such as the Structured Clinical Interview for DSM-IV (Spitzer et al., 1997) or with screening tools such as the MINI-International Neuropsychiatric Interview (Sheehan et al., 1998), the PTSD Checklist (Breslau et al., 1999), the Posttraumatic Diagnostic Scale (Foa et al., 1997), or the Trauma Symptom Inventory (Briere, 1995; Briere et al., 1995).

In addition to assessing for trauma, it is important to assess potential dangers to this patient population. One example of an instrument that has been used with pregnant women in substance use disorder treatment is the Danger Assessment (Campbell, 2007; www.dangerassessment.org). This instrument is a validated measure of the lethality risk women face (Campbell et al., 2009) and can be used to show women the danger they face, as they often minimize this potential, feel worthless, or believe they deserve to be abused. Examples of items that have helped patients understand the severity of danger in their situation include abuse that happens more frequently, abuse that gets rougher (choking, threats of killing her), and hitting her during pregnancy.

STEPS A PROVIDER CAN TAKE TO ASSIST WOMEN IN SEEKING SAFETY FROM ABUSE

There are a number of steps that a provider can take once it is known that a woman is in danger.

Acknowledging the Abuse

The provider should directly and explicitly state that the abuse has happened and is happening and is not right. No one has a right to violate her in this way.

Safety Plan

A safety plan needs to be developed immediately. The provider should ask the patient to identify those in her immediate vicinity (trusted neighbors) or other people she trusts (e.g., family, friends) and develop a code with them for when she is in danger and they should call for help. In preparation for her leaving, which she must do for her safety and the safety of her children, she needs to remove weapons or items that could be used as weapons from the house. She should hide money in a place where she can access it when she leaves. Because the abuser may take her house keys or restrict access to transportation, the provider should strategize with the patient where she can hide an extra set of keys and how transportation could be arranged or negotiated (e.g., a neighbor will drive her to a bus station). A bag with extra clothes and copies of personal documents (e.g., identification card, social security number, health records, etc., and children's records) should be prepared and hidden either in an offsite location or somewhere in the house where the abuser will not discover it.

Any materials that the provider gives the patient should be disguised. For example, phone numbers for safe houses, domestic violence hotlines, trauma support groups, victim services, etc. should not be identified as such. They should be embedded in other material that abusers are not interested in or that look innocuous, such as obstetrical service or educational materials. Finally, only immediately before the woman is leaving should she talk to the children about the departure.

Containment

Plans should be made and strategies should be suggested to the patient for how she can protect herself from further abuse or from an escalation of the abuse.

Support/Affirm

Acknowledge the injustice that has happened to her and emphasize that no one deserves to be treated this way. Affirm that there is hope for the future and that she is not alone in this experience or in leaving this potentially life-threatening situation.

Focus on Coping

Many times providers avoid asking about exposure to violence because they do not know what to do if the answer is "yes." Some providers fear that by discussing the problem they will retraumatize the patient. To lower this risk, rather than asking for details about the abuse or violence exposure, the provider needs to focus on the present situation and the skills the patient can be taught to cope with what has happened and what she can do to avoid future abuse.

Referral

Clinics should have an updated list of referrals to community or national violence exposure services to give to patients. As noted above, any materials given to the patient must be disguised so they do not raise the suspicion of the abuser and risk bringing greater harm to the patient.

TRAUMA-SPECIFIC SERVICES

Trauma-specific services differ from trauma-informed services in that they are designed to treat the actual sequelae of abuse trauma (Jennings, 2004). There are several trauma-specific service models that have been validated through research and are considered best-practice models. The following are models that are widely used in treatment programs for women:

Seeking Safety: A Treatment Manual for PTSD and Substance Abuse (Najavits, 2002; www.seekingsafety.org). The central goal of Seeking Safety is to help patients attain safety from substance abuse; safety from domestic violence and drug-using partners; and safety from extreme symptoms such as dissociation and self-harm (Najavits, 2007). The manual includes handouts and provider guidelines for 25 topics.

Trauma Recovery and Empowerment Model (TREM; Fallot & Harris, 2002; www.ccdc1.org). TREM is a manualized, sequentially organized group approach designed for women with mental health issues, PTSD, and/or substance use disorders. It is co-facilitated by female providers using recovery skills training, psychoeducation, and cognitive-behavioral techniques, with an emphasis on peer support. In addition to the manual, an instructional video is available as well as consultation.

Beyond Trauma: A Healing Journey for Women (Covington, 2003; www.stephaniecovington.com). This program has a specialized curriculum for women's services based on theory, research, and clinical experience. The major emphasis is on coping skills, with specific exercises for developing emotional wellness. There is a facilitator's guide, workbook, and DVD available.

The Sanctuary Model (Bloom, 1994; www.sanctuaryweb.com). This model provides a template for changing the service delivery system to better meet the needs of trauma survivors. It is not directed at patients but at the staff who serve them. It is based on the psychobiology of trauma; the creation of nonviolent environments; principles of social learning; and an understanding of the way systems grow, change, and alter their course. The model was initially developed for use in short-term inpatient psychiatric care for adults traumatized as children. It has been extended for use in multiple settings, including substance abuse programs, domestic violence shelters, and parenting support programs. A manual for implementation of the model and training and consultation services are available.

SUMMARY

A history of trauma is intertwined in the substance use disorders of most women. Treatment providers must ensure that the experience of trauma is core element addressed in the provision of services. Paramount are a safe environment and a culture that recognizes the vulnerabilities of trauma survivors. A history of trauma should be assessed in each patient, as well as current levels of danger. Both trauma-informed services and trauma-specific services must be provided to facilitate engagement in treatment and successful recovery.

REFERENCES

Becker, M. A., Noether, C. D., Larson, M. J., Gatz, M., Brown, V., Heckman, J. P., & Giard, J. (2005). Characteristics of women engaged in treatment for trauma and co-occurring disorders: findings from a national multi-site study. *Journal of Community Psychology*, 33(4), 429–443.

Blanch, A. (2003). *Developing trauma-informed behavioral systems: Report from NTAC's National Experts Meeting on Trauma and Violence*. US Department of Health and Human Services, Substance Abuse and Mental Health Services Administration, Alexandria, VA.

Bloom, S. (1994). The Sanctuary Model: developing generic inpatient programs for the treatment of psychological trauma. In M. B. Williams & J. F. Sommer (Eds.), *Handbook of post-traumatic therapy: a practical guide to intervention, treatment, and research* (pp. 474–491). Westport, CT: Greenwood Publishing.

Breslau, N., Peterson, E. L., Kessler, R. C., & Schultz, L. R. (1999). Short screening scale for DSM-IV posttraumatic stress disorder. *Journal of Psychiatry, 156*, 908–911.

Briere, J. (1995). *Trauma Symptom Inventory professional manual*. Odessa, FL: Psychological Assessment Resources.

Briere, J., Elliott, D., Harris, K., & Cotman, A. (1995). Trauma Symptom Inventory: psychometrics and association with childhood and adult victimization in clinical samples. *Journal of Interpersonal Violence, 10*, 387–401.

Campbell, J. (2007). *Assessing dangerousness: Violence by batterers and child abusers* (Second Edition). New York.

Campbell, J., Webster, D., & Glass, N. (2009). The danger assessment: validation of a lethality risk assessment instrument for intimate partner femicide. *Journal of Interpersonal Violence, 24*, 653–674.

Comfort, M., & Kaltenbach, K. (1999). Biopsychosocial characteristics and treatment outcomes of pregnant cocaine-dependent women in residential and outpatient substance abuse treatment. *Journal of Psychoactive Drugs, 31*(3), 279–289.

Covington, S. (2003). *Beyond trauma: a healing journey for women*. Minnesota: Hazelden.

Covington, S., & Kohen, J. (1984). Women, alcohol, and sexuality. *Advances in Alcohol and Substance Abuse, 4*(1), 41–56.

Fallot, R. D., & Harris, M. (2002). The Trauma Recovery Empowerment Model (TREM): Conceptual and practical issues in a group intervention for women. *Community Mental Health, 38*(6), 475–485.

Foa, E., Cashman, L., Jaycox, L., & Perry, K. (1997). The validation of a self-report measure of posttraumatic stress disorder: the Posttraumatic Diagnostic Scale. *Psychological Assessment, 9*, 445–451.

Harris, M., & Fallot, R. (Eds.) (2001). *New directions for mental health services: Using trauma theory to design service systems*, No. 89. Jossey Bass.

Jennings, A. (2004). *Models for developing trauma-informed behavioral health systems and trauma specific services*. Report prepared for National Technical Assistance Center for State Mental Health Planning (NTAC), National Association of State Mental Health Program Directors (NASMHPD), under contract with the Center for Mental Health Services (DMHS), Substance Abuse and Mental Health Services Administration (SAMHSA), US Department of Health and Human Services.

Killeen T., Hein, D., Campbell, A., Brown, C., Hansen, C., Jiang, H., Kristman-Valente, A., Neuenfeldt, C., Rocz-de la Luz, N., Sampson, R., Suarez-Morales, L., Wells, E., Brigham, G., & Nunes, E. (2008). Adverse events in an integrated trauma-focused intervention for women in community substance treatment. *Journal of Substance Treatment, 35*, 304–311.

Morrissey, J. P., Jackson, E. W., Ellis, A. R., Amaro, H., Brown, V., & Najavits, L. M. (2005). Twelve-month outcomes of trauma informed interventions for women with co-occurring disorders. *Psychiatric Services, 56*(10), 1213–1222.

Najavits, L. M. (2002). *Seeking Safety: a treatment manual for PTSD and substance abuse.* New York: Guilford.

Najavits, L. M. (2007). Seeking safety: an evidence-based model for substance abuse and trauma/PTSD. In K. A. Kiewitz & G. A. Marlat (Eds.), *Therapist's guide to evidence-based relapse prevention: practical resources for the mental health professional* (pp. 141–167). San Diego: Elsevier Press.

Najavits, L. M., Weiss, R. D., & Shaw, S. R. (1997). The link between substance abuse and posttraumatic stress disorder in women: A research review. *American Journal on Addictions, 6,* 273–283.

Sheehan, D. V., Lecrubier, Y., Sheehan, K. H., Amorim, P., Janavs, J., Weiller, E., Herquetta, T., Baker, R., & Dunbar, G. C. (1998). The Mini-International Neuropsychiatric Interview (M.I.N.I): the development and validation of a structured diagnostic psychiatric interview for DSM-IV and ICD-10. *Journal of Clinical Psychiatry, 59,* 22–23.

Spitzer, R. L., Williams, J. B. W., & Gibbon, M. (1997). *Structured clinical interview for DSM-IV-patient version.* New York: Biometrics Research Institute.

Substance Abuse Mental Health Services Administration, National Center for Trauma Informed Care. Available online: www.samhsa.gov/nctic (accessed July 3, 2012).

Teusch, R. (1997). Substance-abusing women and sexual abuse. In S. L. A. Straussner & E. Zelvin (Eds.), *Gender and addictions: men and women in treatment* (pp. 97–122). Northvale, NJ: Jason Aronson.

Velez, M. L., Montoya, I. D., Jansson, L., Walters, V., Svikis, D., Jones, H. E., Chilcoat, H., & Campbell, J. (2006) Exposure to violence among substance-dependent pregnant women and their children. *Journal of Substance Abuse Treatment, 30,* 31–38.

13

Case Management

OVERVIEW

I n this chapter we present case management as an important aspect of care in the comprehensive treatment of drug addiction during pregnancy. We first define case management and review the scope of issues that need to be addressed when treating substance use disorders in pregnant women. Next, we discuss the specific ingredients of a full case management approach for treating substance use disorders in pregnant patients. Finally, the take-home messages from the chapter are summarized.

DEFINITION OF AND INTRODUCTION TO CASE MANAGEMENT

Case management has been defined as a patient-centered group of social service functions that help the patient with multiple needs to access the resources she needs to maintain her drug abstinence (CSAT, 1998; Moxley, 1989). The activities that are part of case management are broad and encompass accessing resources, service linkage, monitoring the success of patient–service linkages, and advocating for the patient to help her meet her needs (CSAP, 1993). There appears to be an expanding demand for case management as a result of the increasingly complex patient care systems and types of problems patient face in their lives (Brindis & Theidon, 1997).

Substance use disorders can precede, coexist with, and/or follow multiple life challenges in a pregnant patient's life. Thus, successful case management must include a comprehensive continuum of services to optimize recovery of the aspects of the patient's life that have been affected by substance use. Such areas for which case management can be helpful (see Chapter 6) include housing, food assistance, linkage to medical care providers (including psychiatrists, general or specialized physicians, and obstetricians), Medicaid benefits, legal assistance for civil or criminal issues, and/or employment or educational services. Other services may also be needed, including child care or parenting assistance. Case management can help create a strength-based scaffolding from which patients can sustain drug abstinence and develop a full life. For pregnant patients, adding case management to effective treatments for substance use disorders such as contingency management (see Chapter 2) has been shown to reduce substance use and reduce needs for services (Jones et al., 2004). Other studies have also demonstrated that case management in the form of home visits, referrals, and transportation has been effective in improving outcomes such as treatment retention, substance use, employment, arrests, incarceration, social support, and birth weight for pregnant women in treatment for substance use disorders (Laken & Ager, 1996; Lanehart et al., 1996). Compared to patients with mental illness, there are fewer empirical studies on case management for patients with substance use disorders to support its effectiveness (e.g., Vanderplasschen et al., 2007). These less-robust findings may be due to a limited range of case management activities within and across substance use treatment programs.

CRITICAL ASPECTS OF CASE MANAGEMENT

Case management is founded upon a core set of ten principles. These principles are adapted from *CSAP's Technical Report 7: Pregnancy and Exposure to Alcohol and Other Drug Use* (CSAP, 1993) and *CSAT Tip 27: Comprehensive Case Management for Substance Abuse Treatment* (CSAT, 1998).

1. Case Management is Comprehensive

The pregnant patient should be understood within the context of her unique life situation, which includes her internal and external issues and her support network. Emphasis is placed on her strengths, although the challenges and potential challenges facing her and the gaps between her needs and her potential are identified as well (CSAP, 1993).

2. Case Management is Coordinated and Continuous

There are many dynamic aspects to case management of a pregnant patient's care when she is being treated for a substance use disorder, and each aspect must be incorporated into an overall strategic plan for service provision. This plan must be as free of gaps as possible (CSAP, 1993).

3. Case Management Involves Active Participation by the Patient

The provider of case management services identifies options for the patient, but the patient must select from the options presented, and then the case manager can help her access the selected services (CSAT, 1998). For example, in filling the unmet need of stable housing, the patient may be asked to choose from a recovery house, a shelter, or a long-term residential treatment setting. The case manager reviews the advantages and disadvantages of each option with the patient, but the patient needs to make her own informed decision. The case manager then helps her access the resources that are needed to act on her decision by giving the patient access to a phone, helping her think about questions that she should ask and that she might be asked, and being available if the facility needs to confirm the patient-given information with a treatment professional.

4. Advocacy Is a Key Component of Case Management

Case management requires advocacy by the patient or on behalf of the patient when dealing with a diverse range of entities, such as families, legal systems, social service agencies, and policymaking groups. Advocacy efforts by the patient or provider include educating the entity about substance use disorders and their treatment and the specific situation or needs of the pregnant patient. Advocacy may entail proactive discussions regarding how a patient might gain access to the service or maintain continued involvement in the service (CSAT, 1998).

5. Case Management Depends Upon Local Community Resources

Case management options and resources depend on what is available in the community where the patient resides.

6. Case Management Is Supportive

In many effective programs, case management is proactively supportive of patients. For example, clinical care providers may escort pregnant patients with substance use disorders to the welfare office or to obtain identification cards needed for securing benefits or employment (Jones et al., 2004). This personal involvement conveys to the patient a level of care and concern. Being familiar with the steps the patient must take to access the service helps the case manager more fully comprehend and appreciate the realities faced by patients and can facilitate the development or revision of appropriate treatment goals (CSAT, 1998).

7. Case Management Is Practical

Typically, the initial focus of case management includes basic survival needs such as food, shelter, and clothing. The next step is to overcome significant barriers to treatment engagement, such as treatment for comorbid psychiatric disorders, lack of transportation, or the need for child care. Helping the patient to establish a plan for meeting her initial needs for survival establishes a positive therapeutic relationship with the patient. Teaching the patient the skills to live a drug-free life and contribute to her family and/or community is an important aspect of case management. These pragmatic skills are taught both by explicit statements and implicit modeling of behavior during interactions between the case manager and the patient (CSAT, 1998).

8. Case Management Is Forward-Thinking

During every phase of treatment, case management should provide the foundation and scaffolding for the next phase of treatment (CSAT, 1998). Every case management activity should build upon the one that preceded it and set the stage for the one that follows it. Each activity should fit into a larger plan developed by the case manager and the patient for initiating and sustaining a drug-free life. This means more than just a life without substance use, but one that also includes multiple rewarding aspects that will cause substance use to be less rewarding.

9. Case Management Is Adaptable

Case management must be able to adapt as the patient's needs change (CSAT, 1998). Pregnant patients with substance use disorders almost always have complex and multifaceted issues. Case management for this population must be flexible so that multiple needs can be addressed concurrently. For example, the patient's health status and case management priorities can change quickly if gestational diabetes is diagnosed. Moreover, some social service agencies are constantly in flux due to tenuous financial or reimbursement status, so priorities may need to be shifted quickly if an agency becomes unable to provide a service.

10. Case Management Is Culturally Sensitive

One of the central features of case management is that it is sensitive not simply to the needs of its patients but also to the need to attend to patient differences. Thus, case management is aware of the diversity of its patients in terms of such factors as age, gender, race, ethnic background, sexual orientation, and physical or mental disabilities.

SPECIFIC INGREDIENTS OF A FULL CASE MANAGEMENT APPROACH

As noted in the chapter introduction, case management is an integral part of a comprehensive treatment for substance use disorders in pregnant patients. The specific activities that make up case management for this population are broad and can be combined in ways specific to the unique needs of each patient. Below we give an overview of many of the activities that are part of a full case management approach.

Intake

At this initial stage of treatment, the staff, especially the case manager and counselor, must quickly establish rapport with the pregnant patient. Fear, mistrust, and reluctance to enter treatment can be overcome by using Motivational Interviewing techniques (see Chapter 2). It is often helpful to provide the patient with neutral, nonjudgmental information about the treatment program, what it provides, and what to expect from each stage of treatment. In this first session, the provider should determine which of the patient's basic needs are unmet and should give initial assistance and provide an overall plan for how the provider and patient can collaborate to meet these needs. Offering a message of hope and empowerment that the patient has the necessary psychological resources to make lasting, positive behavioral changes can help establish a positive rapport. Such a rapport is essential to treatment success.

An important but perhaps tedious part of the intake process is to find out how a patient can be contacted if she does not attend an appointment. Table 13.1 lists elements that have been found to be successful in contacting participants in clinical research studies.

Outreach

Outreach can involve many different levels of intensity and effort. This aspect of care is a challenging one in that, like many other aspects of case management, it is not usually reimbursed by third-party payers. Outreach can be needed for many types of events, such as missed appointments (at the treatment clinic or in another location where the patient has been referred), known lapse to substance use, failure to provide a scheduled urine sample, etc. Typically, outreach should be performed when a patient misses an appointment. Outreach should also be performed when there are reasons to evaluate the patient's health and well-being: perhaps the staff member suspects the patient is being physically abused by a partner or is living in inadequate housing. A successful protocol

Table 13-1. ELEMENTS OF A SUCCESSFUL PATIENT LOCATOR FORM

- Obtain at least three different names of individuals the patient sees regularly and their addresses, phone numbers, pager numbers, e-mail addresses
- For each contact person, ask if the clinic may contact the person by phone, mail, e-mail, and/or home visit
- Nicknames or aliases
- Maiden name
- Locations where the patient "hangs out" during the day
- Locations where the patient "hangs out" during the night
- Place of birth, state and city
- Driver's license number
- Names and addresses, phone number, e-mail addresses, and permission to contact for:
  - Mother
  - Father
  - Social worker
  - Doctor
  - Lawyer
  - Probation or parole officer
  - NA or AA sponsor
  - Place of worship
- Have the patient sign and date the form, attesting to its accuracy
- Review the form with the patient and update it frequently

that has been used in comprehensive care clinics that treat substance use disorders in pregnant women includes starting with telephone contact.

TELEPHONE CONTACT

The patient should be phoned as soon as possible if she fails to appear for her appointment. The phone number called should be the one the patient gave on her intake locator form. Ideally, the person with whom the patient had the appointment should be the caller. Often a semistructured script for this conversation should be used to protect patient confidentiality, and the need to maintain confidentiality should be paramount in the caller's mind.

If the patient is reached by phone, the staff member should express concern that she missed her appointment and should explore the barriers and immediate solutions to those barriers that would allow the patient to complete the appointment the same day (if clinic hours allow). If clinic resources allow, providing transportation will increase the probability that she will attend the appointment. During this conversation with the patient, determining her current location can be helpful if future efforts to locate her are needed.

If the patient is not initially reached by telephone, repeated telephone calls that are documented in the patient's chart should be made for at least two successive days to re-establish contact. It is important to have a phone feature that either blocks or masks the exact phone number and identity of the person and clinic.

LETTERS

Written contact is the next level of intensity for outreach. The use of a standard template that can be individualized for each patient reduces the burden on clinic staff for performing this type of outreach. A letter is sent if the patient cannot be reached by phone or if she fails to visit the clinic following telephone contact. The goal of delivering a letter is to re-engage the patient in treatment. As with telephone communication, confidentiality is of paramount importance. The letterhead should be generic enough that it masks the fact that the clinic is a substance use disorder treatment facility, as well as its exact identity. The letter should either be hand-delivered or mailed to the address or multiple addresses where the patient is known to stay or to other patient-approved contacts listed in the locator form.

Elements of a letter for outreach should include:
- A statement that a specific named person missed seeing her on the specific date the patient did not show up for the appointment
- A statement that we want her to visit the clinic again as soon as possible

- A request to contact the specific person to inform him or her that the patient is doing well or needs assistance
- A closing statement that the clinic and its staff look forward to hearing from her very soon

COMMUNITY VISITS

The highest level of intensity for outreach is the "home visit" or visit to the patient in the community. Home visits should be attempted as soon as the patient shows a pattern of missing appointments. The goal is to bring the patient back to the clinic for the appointment, but when resources allow, the provider performing the outreach should be prepared to conduct an intervention in the community. The goal of the community visit is to re-engage the patient in treatment. This goal has been achieved in programs where the staff member first expresses positive emotions upon seeing the patient, then states that the clinic staff have missed the patient, and finally reminds the patient about her accomplishments to date. The staff member and patient then explore the barriers to and benefits of continued treatment participation, using in a Motivational Interviewing style.

If the patient cannot be found, the staff member should leave a letter for her at the place where she may be most likely to receive it.

Safety procedures must be in place for community visits. Outreach staff members should always leave directions to the location with a point person in the clinic so others know where they are going. They should carry a mobile phone and should call the clinic when they leave the clinic parking lot, when they arrive at the intended location, and then when they are leaving the location. Ideally, two staff members perform the outreach together. Staff members should park in open areas away from alleys or other places where individuals may hide. They should not enter buildings where groups are lingering and should avoid conducting outreach activities after 3 p.m. because data from the FBI's National Incident Reporting System show that on weekdays between 3 and 6 p.m., youth are most likely to engage in crime (Bureau of Justice Statistics, 1991–1993), including gang crime and violence (Snyder & Sickmund, 1997).

Needs Assessment (Initial and Ongoing)

At intake, pregnant women with substance use disorders often display fear and mistrust of any person in authority. The case manager must first win over the patient and find ways to quickly establish trust and built rapport; without trust and rapport, the patient may be lost to treatment. One way to begin establishing a positive relationship is to review the needs the patient has that are not being met and to help her recognize that the provider and agency have resources and connections to empower her to meet those needs. Figure 13.1 shows a checklist of common problems; for each, the patient is asked to rate how much she needs help. Her responses must not be merely collected and then ignored: for each question, there needs to be at least one service to which the patient can be referred. The case manager and the patient should review this list and then rank her needs. This tool can also be used later in treatment to show how much the patient has improved and what issues still need action.

Linking Patients to Appropriate Services

Given the numerous and diverse needs that pregnant patients with substance use disorders have, the process of identifying resources can seem daunting. For clinics without case management staff, it may be less overwhelming to provide case management to these patients if designated staff members within the clinic initiate and maintain relationships with community resources such as civic groups, local and state governmental agencies, nonprofit organizations that focus on one specific need (e.g., a program that helps children become school-ready or provides low-cost day care), other professionals, and the community at large. Developing and maintaining a diverse community network will help ensure appropriate referrals, identify service gaps, expand community resources, and help to address unmet needs. Additional referral sources can be identified by having staff members share their referral sources and experiences and inviting organizations to the clinic to give presentations about their services. The staff member providing the referral must be knowledgeable about the agency to which the patient is being referred. It also helps if the patient has information about the referral process and the consequences of not following through (e.g., "one strike and you're out" or it's okay to miss a few appointments and then receive help). Finally, the staff must pay careful attention to patient confidentiality and must make sure that the appropriate releases are in place before exchanging any information.

Monitoring Match Between Patient and Agency

Just identifying resources for patients is not enough to achieve success in case management: the resources must be frequently evaluated to determine their adequacy and fit for the patient population. Information should be gathered from the referring staff, the agency itself, and the patients who used the service.

DIMENSION	1	2	3	4	PATIENT RATING OF NEED FOR HELP 0 = NO HELP 1 = SOME HELP 2 = MUCH HELP			
					INTAKE	REVIEW	REVIEW	REVIEW
Physical Health								
Prenatal Care	In Care	Occasional	Frequent	Not in Care				
Other Medical Care Needs Specify:___	In Care	Occasional	Frequent	Not in Care				
Other Medical Care Needs Specify:___	In Care	Occasional	Frequent	Not in Care				
Other Medical Care Needs Specify:___	In Care	Occasional	Frequent	Not in Care				
Dental needs	None	Minor	Moderate	Major				
Behavioral/ Psychiatric								
Psychiatric Care Specify problem:___	No History/ no need	In Treatment	Past treatment	Serious				
Psychiatric Care Specify problem:___	No History/ no need	In Treatment	Past treatment	Serious				

Figure 13.1 Maternal Needs Assessment

Parenting skills	No History/ no need	Receiving service	Past treatment	Serious
HIV risk need for HIV prevention skills	No risk/no need	Receiving service	Some past education	Serious need
Family Planning	No History/ no need	Receiving service	Past treatment	Serious
Trauma Recovery	No History/ no need	Receiving service	Past treatment	Serious
Psychosocial				
Transportation	Consistent	Has Access	Irregular	None
Third Party Payor Assistance	Enrolled	Pending	Will Apply	Denied
Support System	Reliable	Questionable	Crisis Only	None
Living Situation	Stable	Fair	Unsafe	Homeless
Communication Skills	Good	Fair	Limited	None
Survival/ Financial				
Employment	Employed	Temporary	Unemployed	Unable
Food	Stable	Adequate	Inadequate	None
Clothing	Stable	Adequate	Inadequate	None
Financial Resources	Stable	Adequate	Inadequate	None
Financial Management	Stable	Adequate	Inadequate	None

Figure 13.1 (Continued)

Postpartum Care

Lactation assistance	No plans to breastfeed	Needs information	Needs consultation	Needs help		
Resources for baby	Stable	Adequate	Inadequate	None		
Birth plan (e.g., type of delivery, postpartum pain management)	Needs to develop	In process	Inadequate	None		
Legal						
Criminal Legal Problems	None	Possible Help needed	Some Assistance	Serious		
Civil Legal Problems (e.g., child custody)	None	Possible Help needed	Some Assistance	Serious		
				Total Score		

Figure 13.1 (Continued)

Advocacy

Advocacy is needed to secure resources for patients not only outside the treatment program, but also inside the program, especially if the program includes many male patients (Brindis & Theidon, 1997). Advocacy not only helps the woman to acquire needed resources but also empowers her to become more assertive and builds a closer relationship with the case manager. However, advocacy cannot stop case managers from fulfilling their legal obligation to report child abuse or neglect or intentions on the part of the patient to harm herself or others.

SUMMARY

Case management is an important component in the overall comprehensive treatment of substance use disorders in pregnant patients. Case management can help establish rapport with the patient. After a patient's basic needs are met, she can then begin to focus on other activities such as finding employment and child care and building drug-free relationships with others that provide the scaffolding for a complete and sustainable drug-free life. Case management for these patients with multiple needs is demanding for the clinic, the staff, and the patient. A full case management approach for pregnant women with substance use disorders includes many components. Staff must be careful to protect the patient's confidentiality when conducting outreach. As demanding as case management can be, it can be very rewarding to watch patients applying their new skills in identifying and selecting resources and then advocating for themselves.

REFERENCES

Brindis, C. D., & Theidon, K. S . (1997). The role of case management in substance abuse treatment services for women and their children. *Journal of Psychoactive Drugs 29*, 79–88.

Bureau of Justice Statistics, FBI National Incident-Based Reporting System, 1991–1993.

Center for Substance Abuse Prevention. (1993). *Pregnancy and exposure to alcohol and other drug use.* CSAP technical report 7. DHHS publication No. (SMA) 93–2040. Rockville, MD: Substance Abuse and Mental Health Services Administration.

Center for Substance Abuse Treatment. (1998). *Comprehensive case management for substance abuse treatment.* Treatment Improvement Protocol (TIP) Series 27. DHHS Publication No. (SMA) 98–3222. Rockville, MD: Substance Abuse and Mental Health Services Administration.

Jones, H. E., Svikis, D., Rosado, J., Tuten, M., & Kulstad, J . (2004). What if they do not want treatment? Lessons learned from intervention studies of non-treatment-seeking drug-using pregnant women. *American Journal on Addictions, 13*, 1–16.

Laken, M. P., & Ager, J. W . (1996). Effects of case management on retention in prenatal substance abuse treatment. *American Journal of Drug Alcohol Abuse, 22*, 439–448.

Lanehart, R. E., Clark, H. B., Rollings, J. P., Haradon, D. K., & Scrivner, L . (1996). The impact of intensive case-managed intervention on substance-using pregnant and postpartum women. *Journal of Substance Abuse Treatment, 8*, 487–495.

Moxley, D . (1989). *The practice of case management. Sage Human Services Guides*, Vol. 58. Newbury Park, CA: Sage.

Snyder, H., & Sickmund, M . (1997). *Juvenile offenders and victims: 1997 update on violence*. Washington, D.C.: U.S. Department of Justice, Office of Juvenile Justice and Delinquency Prevention.

Vanderplasschen, W., Wolf, J., Rapp, R. C., & Broekaert, E. (2007). Effectiveness of different models of case management for substance-abusing populations. *Journal of Psychoactive Drugs, 39*(1), 81–95.

14

Keys to Developing a Comprehensive Care Model

OVERVIEW

This final chapter pulls together, on a macro level, many of the issues we have discussed in prior chapters by presenting how each of the components of assessment and treatment for pregnant patients with substance use disorders can be integrated into a comprehensive care model. Following the introduction, we discuss how to begin developing a comprehensive model; we use the Center for Addiction and Pregnancy in Baltimore, Maryland, USA, as an example of how such a comprehensive program was started and is being maintained. Next, we review the general keys and steps needed for developing a comprehensive care model in a community setting, as well as ways to identify if the process is headed in a less-than-successful direction and how to address issues that might arise. Finally, the take-home points of the chapter are summarized.

INTRODUCTION

To begin developing a model of care for this population, we first need to know the level of care for which it is being developed; for example, is a national, state, county, community, or single hospital model of care? While the model of care discussed in this chapter has been implemented in a single community treatment setting, some of the keys discussed for developing it are universal regardless of the scale of the model.

CASE EXAMPLE

Many comprehensive care models grow out of relationships that have been forged and nourished over years or out of a crisis situation that requires an immediate response from numerous groups. The Center for Addiction and Pregnancy (CAP) was established in response to growing concerns about the long stays some neonates were having in the intensive care unit at the Johns Hopkins Bayview Medical Center hospital. A retrospective record review found that many of these neonates were born to mothers who had evidence of substance use disorders during pregnancy and who had received inadequate prenatal care or substance use treatment. Linkage between obstetrical care and substance use treatment was lacking, and there was no follow-through on referrals from substance use treatment providers for obstetrical care. If patients did enter treatment for their substance use disorder, retention in treatment was poor, and there was evidence that many community substance use treatment facilities did not want to serve this population.

A pilot project that included an obstetrician within a methadone treatment clinic to serve the pregnant patients resulted in improved maternal delivery and infant outcomes compared to what had been observed in patients in treatment for substance use disorders without such onsite obstetrical care. Thus, the pilot program was expanded. CAP was developed through a cooperative agreement between the Johns Hopkins Bayview Medical Center and the State of Maryland Alcohol and Drug Abuse Administration. The State of Maryland Medicaid Administration also provided insights and recommendation (Jansson et al., 1996).

Leaders from the departments of obstetrics, psychiatry, and pediatrics, in cooperation with the state agencies, worked to identify the barriers to care for treating substance use disorders in pregnant women. This task was accomplished by reviewing research data and clinical care records. Experts from outside the geographical area were also brought in to provide advice and guidance on these issues. The main barriers to care that were identified included the need for child care when patients are in treatment, the need for transportation to and from the program, the need for access to friendly and sensitive obstetrical care as well as other medical services, the need to educate the medical community about the issue of substance use disorders in pregnant women, and the need for women-specific treatment services.

CAP's mission was clearly articulated from the inception of the program. It includes reducing the incidence and severity of obstetrical complications, improving birth outcomes while reducing alcohol and substance use, providing family planning services that are acceptable to patients, and ensuring initial and long-term evaluations of children. The target patient population was broadly defined and encompassed pregnant women using alcohol or drugs living in Maryland.

The initial funding for the program was a grant awarded by the State of Maryland. Within 2 years the program was generating a profit for the hospital, largely due to Medicaid funding.

The original program included admitting patients on weekdays within 2 days of the initial contact with the program. The intake assessment included a medical, gynecological, and obstetrical history and a physical examination. A urine toxicology screening for illicit substances was conducted and a breath alcohol test was performed. The Addiction Severity Index (McLellan et al., 1992) was administered to examine problem functioning in the seven domains (medical, legal, employment, alcohol, drug, family/social, and psychiatric) known to be affected by drug addiction. An HIV risk assessment was also undertaken. Each patient was also assigned to an individual counselor who coordinated care for the patient. Later in the program's development, a more formal psychiatric evaluation was incorporated and performed by psychiatric staff.

The program, located on two floors of a hospital campus building, included an assisted living unit staffed 24 hours a day by nursing personnel. This unit was seen as especially important because many of the patients lack stable housing and need medically monitored withdrawal from substances. Typically, patients are admitted to the assisted living unit for 7 nights and then are transferred to the intensive outpatient phase of the program. The assisted living stay also allows patients to experience drug abstinence and facilitates continued drug abstinence once they are transferred to the intensive outpatient level of care.

The intensity of the program decreases as patients gain longer durations of drug abstinence. Patients early in their drug abstinence are typically required to attend treatment 7 days a week for the first month of treatment. If two urine samples (collected once a week on different days without prior notification) are free of drugs and the patient has attended a family support education group, she progresses to attending treatment on weekdays. If she attends regularly and remains abstinent and her psychosocial functioning continues to improve, she can further decrease her attendance based on an individualized schedule set in collaboration with her counselor.

The majority of the counseling is performed in groups. Group topics are tailored to pregnant patients and include psychoeducational groups on obstetrics, Lamaze, family planning, substance use, and occupational assessment. Special therapy groups also exist for patients addressing violence and victimization or patients who need intensive relapse prevention. Patients who desire Twelve Step activities are encouraged to attend meetings in their communities; the program provides help in identifying meetings and sponsors.

One of the keys to success of the CAP model is the open, clear, and transparent communication that takes place both within and across the program units. For example, meetings are held regularly to coordinate care and communication between providers and staff. Each day representatives from the various care units (e.g., intake, nursing, obstetrics, counseling staff, group programming, research, and administration) meet to review the daily attendance records, urine results, admissions, discharges, patients who missed treatment, noncompliant patients, and any staff coverage or other programmatic issues that need attention. At every-other-week meetings more general programmatic issues are discussed with the input of all disciplines of CAP, including psychiatry, obstetrics, pediatrics, and nursing.

There were two preliminary reports on the outcomes of the CAP program using the first 100 patients who delivered with the program while enrolled in treatment (Jansson et al., 1996; Svikis et al., 1997). One report provided descriptive outcomes and the other compared these same outcomes to 46 controls not entering treatment for substance use disorder and showed that as a group, CAP patients had less substance use and higher estimated gestational age at delivery, birth weight, and Apgar scores than did the untreated control group. Infants of CAP patients were also less likely to require neonatal intensive care services; for infants who did require these services, they had, on average, shorter intensive care stays than did the infants of untreated women. When total cost was examined (including substance use treatment), mean net savings associated with CAP treatment was $4,644 per mother–infant pair. This study demonstrated the cost-effectiveness of treatment for drug-abusing pregnant women (Svikis et al., 1997).

This model has faced many challenges since its inception and has undergone several modifications due to changes in reimbursement from third-party payers (Jansson et al., 2007). While the model is not as fully comprehensive as it was initially intended to be, it continues to provide an important service to the community.

STEPS TO DEVELOPING A COMPREHENSIVE
MODEL OF CARE

Key Stakeholders

Key stakeholders, decision makers, and treatment model implementers were involved in developing CAP and defining its mission. Other stakeholders that could be included in such a process are the patients themselves and the many health care and social service providers who encounter women and children in various settings, such as child protective services, welfare workers, social service agency administrators, police, and emergency medical technicians. The views of these individuals are invaluable when developing a comprehensive treatment program. Even if the program is being established at only a single location or institution, this facility may have a far-reaching ability to attract and assist patients from surrounding geographical areas, so having government agencies and leaders on a local or even state level aware and providing input may be critical to the success of the endeavor.

Program initiators must engage community members by soliciting their opinions, building trust, fostering relationships, and participating in community groups. This engagement process will be successful if there is open dialogue and if both the initiators and the community members are willing to exchange ideas. For example, the initiators might establish or join neighborhood community associations, form a task force with residents to solve a particular problem (e.g., reducing loitering at bus stops), or invite community representatives to sit on an internal board, such as an advisory group or a research and development team.

The initiators should also obtain a list of registered organizations from a state or local commission, City Hall, or the courthouse. Organizations with a viable track record and, at a minimum, neighborhood-level membership could be selected for further consideration as possible stakeholders (Fishbein, 1998).

Stakeholder Meetings

Stakeholder meetings are a very expensive endeavor in terms of the cost of labor and what gets accomplished or does not get accomplished in them. Thus, these meetings must be well organized to allow meaningful conversation and dialogue.

First, determine what you want to accomplish in each stakeholder meeting and who should attend. One meeting may be just a meet-and-greet session, getting to know all the various services in the community that serve the pregnant patient population. In that case, you may want the line staff who actually provide the care to give brief introductions about what they do and how they serve the target population. However, if the meet-and-greet is intended to produce buy-in for creating a network of services and producing cooperative agreements between various organizations, you may instead want to invite decision makers or gatekeepers from the various organizations.

Once you decide who should attend the meeting, phone each person to provide him or her with an overview of the goals of the meeting and to convey why it is important for him or her to attend. Follow up the phone calls with an invitation giving the purpose of the meeting, logistical details, the agenda, and a contact person for any questions.

Second, develop the agenda. Ask for input from the attendees or a subset of key attendees. The phone calls made to contact each invitee may provide you with important information that will shape the focus and goals of your meeting. Think carefully about the title of the meeting and each action item because labels can shape the mindset of the attendees. Keep in mind the outcomes you want from the meeting and arrange the agenda so that the activities of the meeting work to reach that outcome. Schedule something important for the beginning part of the meeting to encourage attendees to arrive on time. For each agenda item, include the type of action needed (vote, task outlined and assigned to a person to be done) and the type of product (written document, e-mail, verbal presentation at next meeting, etc.). Give a time estimate for discussing each topic. Ask for commitment to the agenda; if you do not receive it, ask why, and negotiate to get commitment. While the agenda needs to be strategic and structured, it should not be overly planned because this may minimize participant involvement.

Assign someone to record the decisions reached in the meeting and important actions to be taken. This material should be distributed to the attendees within a few days after the conclusion of the meeting.

Third, pay careful attention to the details of how the meeting is conducted. How the meeting is opened sets the stage for the rest of the meeting. Always start the meeting on time. This conveys respect to those who showed up punctually and reminds latecomers that the scheduling is serious. Welcome attendees and thank them for their time. Provide an overview of the agenda, how long the meeting will last, and what the overall goal is for the meeting:

> With the one hour we have today, we have four agenda items to cover: a presentation by community program X, a review of the partnering obstetrical and addiction program relationships already in existence, a summary of the barriers to care in our community, and a decision about what three new stakeholders to invite to the next meeting. Each of these agenda items will help make concrete steps toward our goal of developing a network of care to treat substance use disorders in pregnant women.

Thank and note the person designated to take minutes, and remind the attendees that the minutes with assigned actions and decisions reached will be distributed shortly after the meeting.

The meeting leader must model the type of participation and energy level expected of other attendees. In initial meetings, it is worth considering if the leader's role and the role of each attendee should be reviewed and clarified.

Ensuring the attendees know one another and their respective roles may help to build trust and cohesion in the group.

It may be necessary to set ground rules before the start of the meeting. For example, if confidential information is being shared, it is important to inform attendees that it must not be discussed outside the room or with anyone who did not attend the meeting. Other general rules may include setting a time limit on talking, keeping focused on the agenda topic on the table, not going back to agenda items once they are discussed and completed (a need for closure and firm decisions on items), and requiring active participation. Another effective ground rule is that anyone who raises a problem must also offer a potential solution. Both the ground rules and the agenda should always be visible in every meeting.

Meetings should always be open and transparent. Avoid holding an open meeting followed by a closed meeting.

Often issues arise that are not part of the agenda and are outside of the tasks to be accomplished. Setting the agenda and establishing ground rules will help avoid this common problem. To allow the person to feel "heard" while still keeping the agenda on track, the off-topic ideas can be written in the corner of a whiteboard, and these "parking-lot" ideas can be addressed at the next meeting or briefly discussed at the end of the meeting.

The tone of the meeting should be one of equality and not "we're the outside experts and we're coming in to tell you community members how to do things." Sometimes in a meeting individuals will present a problem to the group or raise a complaint. Two effective ways of addressing their issues are the leader offering a positive perspective of understanding and a solution-focused attitude. For example, conveying through language and actions that "we will be able to solve this issue, and we need to work together to decide how that will happen" may be quite effective in making such attendees feel "heard." When individuals are difficult and present a problem, ask them, "Do you have a recommended solution?" Whenever possible, make these people a part of the solution; influence them to "own" the solution and to take credit for it.

Time management—keeping the momentum of the meeting going, giving each attendee an opportunity to participate and both raise and address issues, and adhering to the agenda—can be difficult. Ways to overcome these issues include managing the decision process rather than the outcome of the decision, using the parking-lot technique, and having a structure to the meeting.

You may want to save 5 to 10 minutes at the end of the meeting to have each attendee evaluate on a scale of 0 = "worst" to 10 = "highest" how useful or effective the meeting was in meeting its goals, or to provide feedback on a specific dimension of the meeting. Seeking feedback from those who rate the meeting low as to how to improve future meetings as well as positive feedback on what went well will be helpful in conducting future meetings and continuing momentum.

End each meeting on a positive note. Summarize the actions and decisions of the meeting, set the time for the next meeting, ask for commitment to attend the meeting, and thank the attendees for their time and participation.

Building Trust Among Stakeholders

Establishing and maintaining trust among stakeholders is vital and takes time, experience, and communication. The development of a comprehensive care model usually begins with one person or a few highly committed and visionary individuals who care deeply about the patient population, want to help them make substantive changes in their lives, and want to improve the way health care providers treat them. Having outside experts come in and provide insight, advice, and expertise about aspects of the model may be helpful, but it should be assumed, unless data have convincingly shown otherwise, that each community has within itself the ability and the tools to heal itself and build a comprehensive care model. Focusing on the model's overarching goals can help remind all stakeholders why everyone is in the room, what needs to be accomplished, and the benefits to both the community and the patient population of creating such a model. Finding common views and goals and focusing on these aspects before moving on to more controversial topics and differences of opinion can be useful for building trust and moving forward in the process.

Strengths and Needs Assessment

Once the stakeholders are identified, conduct an assessment of strengths and needs, such as the most pressing problems in the community, the perceived obstacles and tensions that exist with the community and the target patient group, and proposed resolutions and strategies to solve these issues. Focus on assessing the existing strengths in the community in general as well as strengths specific to the target population. Determine what resources are available to address the issues the population faces (e.g., housing, transportation, child care) and what substance use treatment services exist and are working well. These assets of the community serve as protective factors; that is, they improve residents' resistance to risk factors. Protective factors may include extended families, social cohesion, stable housing, and strong neighborhood groups that currently help or could be mobilized to help the target population.

Stakeholders should fully explore the barriers that keep the target population from obtaining care and remaining in treatment and should formulate strategies to overcome these barriers. The assessment may need to be done over time and with a series of small-group meetings. Once the results of the assessment are known, they should be shared with and evaluated by the stakeholders to provide clear and transparent communication.

The areas of the assessment described above are based on a prevention framework (Substance Abuse and Mental Health Services Administration, 2012a, 2012b) that defines both risk and protective factors in order to direct the problem-solving abilities of the community and the program initiators in tandem. After conducting the needs and strengths assessment, the program developers should understand and be able to engage with the community's resources in general, in addition to the existing substance use treatment services. Having a thorough knowledge of these resources will allow the initiators to build upon them in the comprehensive model for treating substance use disorders in pregnant women.

System-Wide Planning Process

Implementing a comprehensive model of care requires a system-wide integrated strategic planning process that can address the need to create change at every level of the system, ranging from system philosophy, regulations, and funding, to program standards and design, to clinical practice and treatment interventions, to provider competencies and training. An advisory board or steering committee should have input into the system planning and have the authority to define measurable system outcomes and oversee outcomes and continuous quality improvement. However, the board should not direct the oversight of the daily operations of the model.

Formal Consensus On the Model of Care

The system must develop a clear mechanism for articulating the model of care and what it will and will not do. Included should be the principles of treatment and the goals of implementation, developing a formal process for obtaining consensus from all stakeholders, and identifying barriers to implementation and an implementation plan. This information should be distributed to all providers and consumers within the system. Having such a consensus statement will allow for a more unified treatment approach to this patient population and will manage expectations about the responsibilities and roles of services and providers in the model. It is important to document what will be measured and evaluated and how this ongoing evaluation will be done. Part of this process includes the scope of care and defining the separate and intersecting approaches to care that each discipline in the model will bring to the model.

There will probably be considerable common ground upon which consensus can be built, but there will also be areas of disagreement. Through continued conversations and meetings, it will be important to articulate differences and appreciate them as strengths rather than weaknesses.

Coordinating Care Within and Outside of the Model

Implementing the model will involve creating routine structures for staff and providers to communicate and coordinate care within the program. In some cases, they may also need to coordinate with representatives from outside organizations that may participate in caring for complex patients whose needs cross traditional treatment system boundaries. Ideally, these meetings will have both administrative and clinical leadership and will be designed not just to solve particular clinical problems, but also to foster a larger sense of shared clinical responsibility throughout the service system. These meetings should be designed to build bridges and foster interdependence. An outcome of this process may include the development of specific policies and procedures formally defining the mechanisms by which obstetrical and addiction treatment providers support one another and participate in collaborative treatment planning, conflict resolution, and coordination of ongoing care for substance use disorders in pregnant patients.

Developing Basic Dual-Diagnosis Competencies

Treating pregnant patients with substance use disorders requires competencies in terms of providers' attitudes, values, knowledge, and skills. A listing of available provider competencies for prenatal care and substance use disorder treatment can be used as a reference point for beginning to build both consensus and trust regarding competencies among the various providers and agencies. Mechanisms must be developed to establish the competencies in existing human resource policies and job descriptions; to incorporate them into personnel evaluation, credentialing, and licensure; and to measure or monitor provider attainment of competency. Existing competency assessment measures may need to be modified to facilitate this process. This modification process of assessment of competencies will need input from outside experts knowledgeable about the rules and regulations of each discipline. There should be an emphasis on understanding what all the other providers are doing while maintaining each provider's individual scope of practice.

System-Wide Training Plan

In any comprehensive care model, training of professionals treating the patients must be ongoing and tied to expected competencies in the context of actual job performance. This goal requires an organized training plan to bring training and supervision to both prenatal care providers and substance use treatment providers on site. The most common components of such training plans are curriculum development and dissemination, mechanisms for training and deploying trainers, career ladders for advanced certification, and opportunities for experiential learning.

Peer Recovery Supports

Many well-coordinated comprehensive care programs offer self-help programs, access to Twelve Step programs, and peer-support mentors or Big Sister programs. Having a plan to establish these peer-to-peer help groups or networks and carefully monitoring them to make sure they are therapeutic can be a decided benefit to the success of the overall model of care. Recovery-oriented systems of care (SAMHSA, 2009) have also identified the use of peer recovery support specialists (persons in recovery who have been trained and certified to work as paid staff in behavioral health) as important components of peer recovery support.

COMMON STUMBLING BLOCKS

One of the stumbling blocks that inhibit communities from building a comprehensive care model for treating substance use disorders during pregnancy is that it can seem overwhelming to bring together so many different people from so many different organizations with differing and sometimes competing viewpoints. It can also seem quite expensive, especially if there is the assumption that many services will need to be offered, such as those provided at CAP. However, there are ways to overcome these issues.

Start small. Focus on bringing a few like-minded, committed providers together. Develop a pilot project like the one described above, where the director of the methadone maintenance program had an obstetrician who was willing to come to the methadone clinic a day or two a week and provide prenatal care to the methadone-maintained women. This brought only two of the components together, but it improved care in a meaningful way and generated data to support an expanded effort. Starting with a small and specific collaboration of two programs allows for processes to be tested and problems that arise to be ironed out before implementing the program on a larger scale. Given the extreme pressure many obstetricians are under in terms of liability insurance and the need for high patient volumes to offset a low reimbursement rate, it may be difficult to find a provider willing to travel offsite. Thus, having a solid linkage program where the patient receives transportation to and from the obstetrics clinic, along with good communication and coordination of services between the methadone provider physician and the obstetrician, can also be the start of a comprehensive care model. Information on programs and services that address the multiple issues pregnant patients with substance use disorders face can be shared between the programs.

Conflicting approaches toward care can be another stumbling block that comprehensive care model developers face. Even terminology can reflect these differing philosophies in the approach to care: some care models use the term "patient" to describe the individual being treated, but others use "client." Some see "client" as an empowering term, whereas "patient" implies giving up one's power to a medical professional. To the best of our knowledge, there are no data to support the use of one word over the other in terms of outcomes for substance use treatment. One survey of psychiatric patients showed that 77% of them preferred to be called "patients" rather than "clients" (Ritchie et al., 2000). One way to resolve this issue is to ask each woman which term she prefers (Wing, 1997).

Differing philosophies can also be reflected in such aspects of care as the degree to which there is the need for treatment to be voluntary, the need for informed consent to care, the provision of continued care based upon adherence to all aspects of care, the use and necessity of medications to treat illnesses, and the urgency with which care should be provided. When addressing the conflicts that arise due to differing philosophies of treatment, it is important to remember that providers share the same goal of a successful outcome for the pregnant woman with a substance use disorder. Where possible, the discussion should be focused on finding common ground and identifying and implementing solutions to problems, at the same time respecting the fact that the differing philosophies of care exist.

As technology advances, the competing interests of the mother and the provider may be at odds. The risks and benefits for mother, her fetus, and the mother–fetus dyad must be carefully discussed and weighed in discussions between the provider and patient (Jones, Finnegan, & Kaltenbach, 2012; Jones et al., 2012).

PRINCIPLES OF THE MODEL

For a comprehensive care model to succeed, the community needs to address the underlying problems that lead to drug addiction and the way in which patients are treated by the community. Conversely, it is also important for patients to recognize their responsibilities in participating in the larger community.

The comprehensive care model requires comprehensive strategies for addressing the multiple issues of the pregnant patient. Substance use treatment programs appear to achieve the best outcomes for their patients when they have the active participation of a multidisciplinary team of individuals capable of thoroughly assessing problems, treating them, and preventing future ones from arising.

Principles of treatment must be agreed upon by the care providers. As described above, it can be challenging to develop a comprehensive care model when there are two competing philosophical approaches to care. Thus, for a program to be successful, some agreed-upon principles of treatments need to be explicitly stated. For example:

1. Belief that empathic, hopeful, and integrated treatment relationships are one of the most important contributors to treatment success in any setting. As discussed in Chapter 3, the use of accurate empathy is a powerful and effective ingredient in the therapeutic relationship. Thus, a comprehensive care model needs to establish clear guidelines for how providers in any service setting can provide integrated treatment in the context of an appropriate scope of practice. Using this common belief, agreement needs to be found and clear guidelines written for providers and staff that outline how patients should access care and what the guidelines are for continuing to receive this integrated care.

2. Agreement that the guidelines that are most proactive and conservative will be used as the guiding principles of model operation. For example, in the case of patient confidentiality, the more conservative rule of making patient confidentiality of paramount importance will be used. The guideline that medical providers cannot ethically wait to treat a patient when her functioning is actively deteriorating is another guiding principle (of course, an operational definition of what level of deterioration is acceptable before intervening must be established to avoid conflict within a treatment team). Clearly establishing the

expectations and responsibilities of each care provider with the patient
as well as the expectations and responsibilities of the patient can
help alleviate conflicts in the comprehensive care relationships. For
example, one issue that repeatedly arises in comprehensive substance
use treatment models for pregnant women is the issue of if and how
prenatal care should be continued if the patient is not attending
substance use treatment as agreed upon by the treatment provider
and patient. One way to address this issue is to have the patient sign a
behavioral contract indicating that the prenatal care will be continued
but only at a specific time so that the patient can be discharged
from substance use treatment and not be onsite at the clinic during
the regular substance use treatment times. To address the concern
that providers are "throwing patients out of treatment," there can
be clear guidelines for how much time the patient must wait and/or
those activities the patient must complete in order to be eligible for
readmission to the substance use treatment program.

3. Both the health of the pregnancy and treatment of the substance
disorder should be considered primary, and integrated treatment is
recommended. The model is treating patients for both prenatal care
and substance use disorders, and neither one should take primary
focus. The system needs to develop a variety of administrative,
financial, and clinical structures to reinforce this clinical principle,
and specific practice guidelines should emphasize how to integrate
these two conditions needing care using the best practice treatments
appropriate for patients within each service.

SUMMARY

Developing a comprehensive care model takes time, practice, and a high level of
dedication. The initiators must have a vision of how treatment of the pregnant
patient with substance use disorders can improve her life and the lives of her
future children. To establish a comprehensive care model, the initiators must
hold meetings of the various stakeholders and engage them in constant and
ongoing communication so that a clear consensus about the approach to caring
for this population can be developed. The model can start with a few essential
components and be gradually expanded. While there are often differences of
opinion over philosophies of care, it is important to find common ground and
have procedures for care, communication, and resolution of the conflicts that
inevitably arise between and among disciplines. The illness of substance use

disorders takes time to develop, and the situation becomes even more complex when the patient is pregnant. Thus, this disorder requires an equally complex and comprehensive treatment response.

REFERENCES

Fishbein, D. (1998, May). *The comprehensive care model—citizen participation in crime prevention.* Presented by the FBI Law Enforcement Bulletin.

Jansson, L. M., Svikis, D., Lee, J., Paluzzi, P., Rutigliano, P., & Hackerman, F. (1996). Pregnancy and addiction. A comprehensive care model. *J Substance Abuse Treatment, 13*(4), 321–329.

Jansson, L. M., Svikis, D. S., Velez, M., Fitzgerald, E., & Jones, H. E. (2007). The impact of managed care on drug-dependent pregnant and postpartum women and their children. *Substance Use and Misuse, 42*(6), 961–974.

Jones, H. E., Finnegan, L. P., & Kaltenbach, K. (2012). Methadone and buprenorphine for the management of opioid dependence in pregnancy. *Drugs, 72*(6), 747–757.

Jones, H. E., Kaltenbach, K., Heil, S. H., Stine, S. M., Coyle, M. G., Arria, A. M., O'Grady, K. E., Selby, P., Martin, P. R., Jansson, L., & Fischer, G. (2012). Intrauterine abstinence syndrome (IAS) during buprenorphine inductions and methadone tapers: can we assure the safety of the fetus? *Journal of Maternal-Fetal and Neonatal Medicine, 25*(7), 1197–1201.

McLellan, A. T., Kushner, H., Metzger, D., Peters, R., Smith, I., Grissom, G., Pettinati, H., & Argeriou, M. (1992). The Fifth Edition of the Addiction Severity Index. *Journal of Substance Abuse Treatment, 9*(3), 199–213.

Ritchie, C. W., Hayes, D., & Ames, D. J. (2000). Patient or client? The opinions of people attending a psychiatric clinic. *Psychiatric Bulletin, 24*, 447–450.

Substance Abuse and Mental Health Services Administration. (2009). *What are peer recovery support services?* Washington, DC: Publication SMA09-4454.

Substance Abuse and Mental Health Services Administration. (2012a). *Prevention of substance abuse and mental illness.* Available online: http://captus.samhsa.gov/prevention-practice/strategic-prevention-framework (accessed July 1, 2012).

Substance Abuse and Mental Health Services Administration. (2012b). *Recovery-oriented systems of care.* Available at: http://partnersforrecovery.samhsa.gov (accessed July 23, 2012).

Svikis, D. S., Golden, A. S., Huggins, G. R., Pickens, R. W., McCaul, M. E., Velez, M. L., Rosendale, C. T., Brooner, R. K., Gazaway, P. M., Stitzer, M. L., & Ball, C. E. (1997). Cost-effectiveness of treatment for drug-abusing pregnant women. *Drug and Alcohol Dependence, 45*(1–2), 105–113.

Wing, P. C. (1997). Patient or client? If in doubt, ask. *Canadian Medical Association Journal, 157*, 287–289.

INDEX